The confident

girl's guide

to a

leak-free

life

3rd Edition

Mary O'Dwyer

Women's Health Physiotherapist

HOLD IT SISTER
THE CONFIDENT GIRL'S GUIDE TO A LEAK-FREE LIFE
Third Edition
Copyright © 2011 MARY O'DWYER

First published in 2007 as 'My Pelvic Flaw' and revised 2008,
Published as 'Hold it Sister' 2009, 2010 (2nd Ed)
RedSok Publishing
PO Box 1881, Buderim, Queensland, Australia 4556
www.redsok.com

www.holditsister.com

National Library of Australia Cataloguing-in-Publication Data
O'Dwyer, Mary Rose.
  Hold it Sister: the confident girl's guide to a leak-free life
  Bibliography.
  1. Pelvic floor--Care and hygiene
  2. Pelvic floor--Health aspects
  3. Pelvic floor--Diseases--Prevention
  4. Pelvic floor--Diseases--Treatment
  Dewey Number: 617.55

ISBN: 978-0-9870766-0-1

Cover Design & Illustrations by Maggie Allingham
Edited by Tania McCartney,
Photography by Barry Alsop, Eyes Wide Open

Disclaimer
All names used in the case studies are fictional. This book represents research and clinical experience, is for educational use and is designed to help the reader make informed decisions.
This book is not a substitute for treatment by a physiotherapist or doctor.
The publisher, author and distributors expressly disclaim any liability to any person for any injury or inconvenience sustained, or for any use or misuse of any information contained in this book. The author has made every effort to provide accurate and clear information in the book, and cannot be responsible for any misinformation.

This book is a work of non-fiction. The author asserts her moral rights.

About the Author

Mary O'Dwyer is an Australian women's health physiotherapist who trained at the Universities of Queensland and Melbourne. With over thirty years clinical experience and consulting in women's health, she is now an international teacher and author alongside her role as a Senior Teaching Fellow at Bond University.

Mary conducts practical and informative one-day workshops for women and delivers workshops for fitness professionals, teaching safe training strategies to prevent pelvic floor problems related to over-challenging exercise. Mary has become an advocate for introducing new assessment protocols and safe exercise guidelines into the Fitness Industry to identify and protect women with, or at risk of developing, pelvic floor dysfunction.

Having witnessed the effects of pelvic floor dysfunction from her patients' stories, Mary is committed to educating women about their pelvic health, and to enlighten and empower them in the management of relevant problems, while giving them the confidence to make informed decisions.

Hoping to reach more women than her professional practice allows, 'Hold it Sister' is set to transform women's knowledge of their pelvic floor and its central role in the female body.

Contents

5. Pregnancy, Birth and Postpartum

6. Menopause and the Pelvic Floor

7. Taking Action

Hamlin Foundation

**Ten per cent of the profits from the sale
of this book will be donated to:**

The Hamlin Foundation for
Fistula Surgery in Ethiopia

After witnessing horrific injuries suffered by African women in childbirth, Dr Catherine and Dr Reg Hamlin commenced surgery in Addis Ababa in the 1960s. The affected women suffer extensive internal damage through birthing babies too large for their pelvis. The resulting damage leaves them unable to control the flow of urine or faeces. This in turn leads to rejection by their family, forcing them to live as destitute outcasts from their villages.

Surgery and care at a Fistula Hospital repairs the damage, restoring the women's dignity, allowing most of them to return to their homes.

To learn more, visit www.fistulatrust.org

'Over the course of a lifetime, one in 30,000 Scandinavian women dies in pregnancy or labour. For a woman from Africa, the risk is one in 12. However, for every woman who dies in labour in the developing world, many more find their lives destroyed by terrible injuries because of untreated obstructed labour. The developed world is only now becoming aware
of the devastation to women's lives, largely because women in the developing world have no voice in the international community'.

– International Continence Society -

The Pelvic Floor

1

Our Pelvic Flaw

The female pelvic floor responds and greatly benefits through practising effective daily habits and specific exercise to ensure it continues to function with peak efficiency throughout life. Female pelvic floor dysfunction is too often accepted as part of 'being female', with many women embarrassed to speak to family or partners when problems occur. Unfortunately, the pelvic floor remains a mystery to most women, so years of ongoing dysfunction are endured before seeking help.

Through my clinical work, it became obvious women wanted easily understood information to help them protect this precious body area from damage associated with poor daily habits, over challenging exercise, childbirth, and the effects of menopause and ageing. They told me their pelvic floor problems and resultant poor quality of life were not acceptable and later became passionate advocates for spreading information to daughters and friends. 'Hold It Sister' evolved over a decade of hearing women ask 'Why didn't some one tell us this information before?' The information in this book will empower women with practical skills to protect or improve their pelvic floor function. It also includes research based knowledge to give confidence when discussing treatment options with health care professionals.

Improved pelvic health long term involves recognising any barriers in the form of damaging habits or activities. I have listed examples of these and the healthy habits to replace them. Also included are practical sessions to reinforce correct learning of the pelvic floor muscle action and I strongly recommend you take the time to do these as you work through the book. Specific advice for pregnancy, birth preparation and postpartum recovery is included with guidelines on returning to activity after baby is born. As pelvic organ prolapse affects 50 per cent of childbearing women, the causes, prevention, and treatment options are discussed. Guidelines for exercising during the menopausal years and overcoming hormonal pelvic floor changes are also included.

I hope you personally apply this knowledge, teach your daughters and talk to other women in order to prevent unnecessary pelvic floor dysfunction and help restore quality of life.

This book is based on my clinical knowledge and the findings of researchers. It should be used as an adjunct to consultations with women's health physiotherapists and medical specialists rather than a substitute. My thanks go to so many wonderful women for urging and inspiring me to write this book; to my colleagues for their encouragement; to my ever-patient husband for his constant support and professional assistance and to the multitude of researchers whose findings underpin my clinical work.

> *Following advice in this book and making changes to lifestyle habits, exercise methods, nutrition, lifting techniques, and toileting strategies will make a huge difference to your quality of life.*

What is the Pelvic Floor?

The pelvic floor is an intriguingly complex area with a span of muscles, tendons, nerves, blood vessels, ligaments and fascia (a tough inter-connecting membrane). It contains different layers, namely the endopelvic fascia, the levator ani muscles, the perineal membrane and the external genitals. The muscles sit in the base of the pelvic girdle bones, which join at the pubic symphysis in front and at the sacro-iliac joints in the back (Fig. 1).

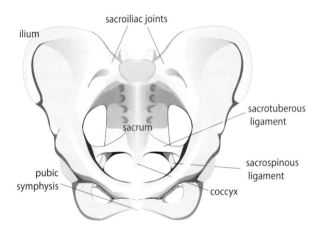

Fig. 1 - Pelvic Girdle Bones from above

The pelvic floor muscles (PF muscles) attach underneath the pubic bone and join into the pelvic sidewalls, sitting bones and the coccyx bone at the base of the spine. Think of them as muscles in a bowl shape, with a trampoline-like action providing 'lift and hold' for pelvic organs to close sphincters and prevent loss of fluid, wind and solids (Fig. 2 & 3). Just as a trampoline lifts on recoil, these muscles can be voluntarily

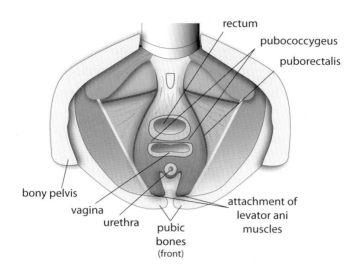

Fig. 2 - Pelvic Floor, from above

lifted (known as the 'knack'), before the additional load of sneezing, running or lifting a weight.

The Incredible Pelvic Floor Muscles

These 'down under' muscles are unrecognised, multi tasking achievers, thanklessly coordinating various tasks every day of your life. Many women are not comfortable discussing pelvic floor problems or mistakenly believe these problems are a normal part of ageing. Understanding the multiple actions of the pelvic floor will reinforce the need for regular attention to maintain good pelvic health.

The role of healthy PF muscles in maintaining continence, preventing internal organ descent, enhancing sexual pleasure, supporting the growing uterus, and working with other muscles to support the spine and pelvis is discussed below.

1. Maintain Continence

The pelvic floor muscles are designed to close and reinforce the sphincters of your bladder and bowel, preventing loss of fluids, wind and solids during movement, sneezing or exercise.

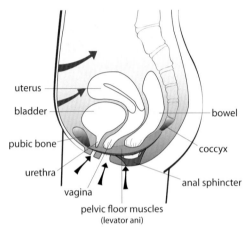

uterus

bladder

bowel

pubic bone

coccyx

urethra

anal sphincter

vagina

pelvic floor muscles
(levator ani)

The levator ani muscles contract to close
the urethral and anal sphincters and draw
up the vaginal walls

Fig. 3 – Pelvic Floor Elevation

2. Protect the Spine

The PF muscles do not work alone. They tighten with the deep abdominal muscle (transversus abdominis), diaphragm and deep spinal muscles (multifidus). Think of PF muscles as the queen of your core muscles. When they tighten and lift, the deep 'core' abdominal and deep spinal muscles automatically tighten in unison. In conjunction with the strong trunk muscles, they support the spine to prevent injury during activity.

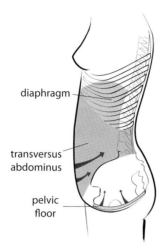

diaphragm

transversus
abdominus

pelvic
floor

The action of pelvic floor and transversus is
to tension and brace against downward
internal pressure.

Fig. 4 – Inner Cylinder of 'Core' Muscles

3. Support the Pelvic Organs

The healthy pelvic floor automatically lifts and holds to support
the bladder, uterus and bowel during activity. Pelvic organ
prolapse occurs when the pelvic organs descend and bulge
down into the vaginal walls. Prolapse is common in women
and prevention relies on practicing correct pelvic floor habits
and maintaining PF muscle strength throughout life. (Refer to
prolapse on page 124).

4. Contribute to Sexual Sensation

During orgasm, PF muscles contribute to sexual sensation and
the intensity of muscle contraction. Rhythmic contractions
occur in the pubococcygeus muscle (PC) and other PF
muscles along with contractions of the anal sphincter,
rectum, perineum, fallopian tubes, uterus and vagina. Strong,

responsive PF muscles maintain vaginal wall strength and orgasmic sensation.

5. Open for Childbirth and Elimination

During crowning, as baby's head moves down through the pelvic floor, relaxation without tightening reduces the risk of muscle tearing. Relaxation of the pelvic floor also facilitates full bladder and bowel emptying.

What Causes Pelvic Floor Problems?

It is a common myth that childbirth is the sole cause of pelvic floor problems. While giving birth contributes to pelvic floor dysfunction in some women, many other factors contribute to the variety of symptoms indicating all is not well 'down under'. The main causes of problems and their symptoms are explained in this section.

Pelvic Floor Muscle Weakness

Signs of weakness include:

- Leaking urine with sneezing, orgasm, lifting or exercise (stress incontinence).
- Frequent toileting 'just in case' (this habit trains the bladder to only hold smaller volumes of urine).
- Rushing to get to the toilet quickly and perhaps leaking urine on the way (urge incontinence).
- Poor control of wind or bowel contents (faecal incontinence), urgency or feeling the bowel has not fully emptied.
- Bulging at the vaginal entrance, a heavy dragging

sensation, pelvic and sexual pain, indicates the organs have slipped down into the vaginal walls (pelvic organ prolapse).

- Loss of vaginal sensation and orgasm strength.

Pelvic Floor Muscle Tightness

Signs of tightness include:

- Bladder urgency and straining to pass urine; perhaps with frequent voiding and passing small amounts of urine.
- Constipation, straining, anal fissures and haemorrhoids.
- Pain with sexual penetration or insertion of tampons.
- Trigger points in internal and external pelvic muscles.
- Altered breathing patterns and excessive abdominal and PF muscle tension.

Constipation

Straining to open the bowel progressively damages the nerves supplying PF muscles, causing a loss of bladder and bowel control. Chronic straining weakens bladder, uterine or bowel supports and contributes to prolapse. Delayed or incomplete emptying is typically due to prolapse of the back (posterior) vaginal wall or failure to release the anal sphincter.

Waist Measurement

Women with a larger waist measurement have a higher risk of pelvic floor dysfunction. Visceral fat accumulates internally around the pelvic organs making PF muscles work harder to support the weighted organs. Visceral fat acts like an endocrine gland releasing chemicals which weaken the ability of connective tissues to recover after damage, e.g. after childbirth or prolapse surgery. Overweight incontinent women show significant improvement of their continence when they lose weight. Research shows a diet high in calories and saturated fat (found in cream, cheese, processed meats, fried food) causes a 2.5 times increased risk of incontinence in women, possibly due to the inflammatory effect created in the body by the higher saturated food intake.

Lifting

The internal abdominal pressure created by heavy lifting overwhelms pelvic floor control when the muscles lack a quick, strong, coordinated lift and hold. If PF muscles fail to lift and hold during heavy tasks, internal supporting ligaments are at risk of being stretched, leading to pelvic organ prolapse.

Pregnancy and Childbirth

Pelvic joints and ligaments are under strain during pregnancy due to the extra load of baby and amniotic fluid.

The use of forceps or ventouse (vacuum extraction) to assist birth is associated with a higher rate of damage to pelvic floor muscles and tendons. Just as damaged muscles, tendons and ligaments are rehabilitated after falls, surgery or sport; the pelvic floor also responds to an effective programme of strengthening pre and postpartum.

Studies show pregnant women are at more risk of developing ongoing postpartum stress incontinence when they experience any of the following factors: urge incontinence before pregnancy, incontinence during pregnancy, a rapid birth or second stage delay in labour, the baby's birth weight is over 4 kg or the baby has a large head. A pre pregnancy maternal body mass index (BMI) exceeding 25 is also a risk factor. BMI is a measure of body composition and can be calculated at the following site: www.nhlbisupport.com/bmi

Over Challenging Exercise

The pelvic floor is a smaller muscle group that is rarely trained to counter the internal forces created with activity, and during exercise will often fatigue long before the heart or lungs. The endurance required for a long run, or prolonged exercise is considerable, and damage occurs when the pelvic floor fatigues part way through a workout. Building abdominal strength with isolated bracing exercises increases intra abdominal pressure with the potential to overwhelm pelvic floor control. Repeated rises of intra-abdominal pressure or even one sudden, heavy episode may result in pelvic floor damage, even prolapse, in some women. If continued fast or high-load exercise results in loss of PF and core muscle control, other muscles substitute to provide trunk stability. Over time the body adopts incorrect muscle substitution, movement patterns and altered posture when the PF and core muscles repeatedly fail in their roles of strength and endurance.

Returning to exercise or lifting heavy weights before regaining PF muscle strength and postural alignment postpartum, results in more strain and damage to pre-weakened muscle, supporting ligaments and connective tissue supports.

Conversely, sustained vigorous exercise (without rest periods) in some women results in increased PF muscle tone causing continued over activity in their PF muscles. Poor bladder and bowel control, painful intercourse and some pelvic pain syndromes are due to increased resting tone (tightness) in PF muscles. Muscular hyperactivity during exercise is avoided by building in regular relaxation breaks and modifying over challenging exercise or training programmes.

Prolonged Coughing

Women with chronic lung or respiratory disorders (asthma, cystic fibrosis, bronchitis) or who smoke, have a higher rate of stress incontinence. Lifting up PF muscles, the 'knack,' before coughing helps prevent urine loss and pelvic organ prolapse.

Weak Connective Tissue

Collagen is the protein in connective tissue giving strength to skin, joints, muscles, ligaments and tendons. Studies indicate when a mother experiences prolapse, daughters have a higher risk of future prolapse.

Hypermobile joints (knees, elbows, fingers and thumbs that bend too far backwards) due to joint laxity and soft tissue elasticity, are a predicator of a higher risk of prolapse following childbirth. It is important for mums with hypermobile joints to focus on PF exercises, adopt protective habits and discuss birthing options with their midwife and doctor. For more information: www.hypermobility.org

Emotional Reactions

Just as some people unconsciously clench their jaws and grind their teeth with tension, others unknowingly store 'emotional' tension in PF muscles. When these muscles are constantly held tight, the resulting pattern of excess tension causes bladder and bowel dysfunction and pelvic pain. Effective treatment involves a program of breathing training, relaxation techniques, muscle stretches, soft tissue mobilization and specific PF exercises. In addition to treating physical symptoms, professional counselling assists with recognition of underlying causes of tension.

Why is Pelvic Floor Dysfunction a Problem?

While pelvic floor dysfunction may be no more than a nuisance to some women, others find it increasingly affects their quality of life.

- Many women restrict activity or sport and stop exercise, fearing urine loss or aggravation of an existing prolapse. Resultant weight gain due to inactivity increases pressure down onto the pelvic floor.

- Some women become isolated, afraid to venture far from home, missing social and travel opportunities.

- Frequent toilet visits at night disturb normal sleep patterns, causing fatigue during the day and increasing the risk of falls in older women.

- When sexual dysfunction is present (poor sensation, weak orgasm, pain or losing urine during sex), relationships suffer through loss of intimacy.

- Chronic pelvic pain contributes to depression and negative thinking. Holding PF muscles tight due to anxiety, stress, trauma, pain or fear, produces painful trigger points in the muscles.

- The expense of buying pads and medication is a hidden

cost of incontinence and a financial burden to women, especially those on a limited income.

There is no one particular treatment for all pelvic floor problems. A woman with a weak pelvic floor will benefit from strength training. A woman with a tight, painful pelvic floor will benefit from initally learning muscle relaxation. Strength training would cause muscle spasms and intensify her pelvic floor pain. Another woman might substitute stronger abdominal and buttock muscles for the pelvic floor action, and will benefit from learning the coordinated lift of PF muscles with core and abdominal muscles first, before strengthening.

Accurate identification of any dysfunction is critical to ensure the correct therapy. Complete the practical activities in this book to understand how your pelvic floor works. You will identify any barriers preventing your PF muscles from working effectively, and then progress through the steps towards regaining control.

Pelvic Floor Habits

2

Five Healthy Pelvic Floor Habits

1. Try a New Toilet Position

Before Thomas Crapper introduced the toilet to nineteenth-century London, squatting was the position commonly used to empty the bowel. Squatting positions the rectum for more complete emptying.

If your habit is to slump and strain, you are at risk of aggravating bladder incontinence, rectal and/or vaginal prolapse.

Start adopting this new position to reduce pelvic floor strain.

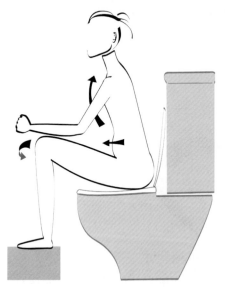

Toilet Position:

- Place your feet on a stool, rest forearms on thighs.
- Straighten your lower back by growing tall.
- Open your knees and lean forward from your hips (keeping your chest up).
- Breathe deeply – open abdomen and base of ribs – and totally relax your abdomen forwards.

Fig. 5. - Correct Toilet Position

Avoid slumping your spine, bearing down or drawing your waist backwards, as these actions close the anal sphincter. A relaxed sphincter promotes efficient bowel emptying.

When the bowel signals it is time to empty, don't put off the urge for too long as this leads to constipation. Establish a regular time for bowel emptying; relax and avoid rushing due to a busy schedule. Stress causes abdominal tension, which makes bowel emptying more difficult and promotes straining.

If you have a slower emptying bowel, look at:

- increasing dietary fibre levels
- increasing water intake
- starting regular exercise
- adopting the new toilet position with waist relaxation

While washing hands after toileting, tighten the anal sphincter and lift up through the back passage. Hold this action and breathe for 5–10 seconds.

For more information: www.aboutconstipation.org

After pelvic repair surgery or childbirth, protect the pelvic floor during bowel opening. Wrap toilet paper around your hand, using it to support the vaginal area as the bowel opens.

When the bowel contents are soft but still not emptying, the cause may be a back vaginal wall prolapse. Sometimes, thumb pressure applied internally to the back vaginal wall is needed to assist emptying.

Ongoing constipation and emptying problems require review by a gynaecologist and women's health physiotherapist.

Case Study

Eileen, a 29 year-old bank manager, was referred by her gastroenterologist for a pelvic floor program. Her habit of straining since childhood had caused her bowel to prolapse forwards into the back of her vaginal wall. She had no children. Examination of Eileen's food and fluid diary showed she ate around 15 grams of fibre (30-35 grams is required daily for a soft bowel motion) and drank only one glass of water (she mostly drank coffee or soft drink). Eileen worked long hours and gave no priority to her need for regular exercise.

To empty her bowel Eileen slumped, strongly pulled her waist back and strained down firmly onto a tight anal sphincter. This was her pattern of toileting since childhood.

Eileen began a new routine of drinking six glasses of water daily, eating fruit or vegetables with every meal and adding whole grains along with a daily fibre supplement to her diet. She started a walking program, PF exercises and adopted (for life) the correct toileting position and abdominal relaxation for easier bowel emptying.

At her third visit, Eileen was delighted to report her bowel was opening, without straining, every second day instead of once every six days.

2. Improve Your Posture

Try this activity to reinforce why tall posture is an essential daily habit to maintain pelvic floor and core muscle activity. Sit on the edge of your chair and become aware of what happens to your pelvic floor with changes of position. Go into a full slump, then grow tall through the crown of your head. Try this action again and feel how the pelvic floor relaxes during the slump then lightly firms when you sit tall *without any apparent effort to actively contract these muscles*. What a powerful incentive to stay tall when sitting and standing.

Be smarter in the chairs you choose to support your spine. Best choice is a straight-backed chair with support up to, but below, the shoulder blades. Lounge chairs with a high headrest push the spine into a slumped or 'C' curved position. Keep both feet flat on the floor with knees relaxed. When your back tires, place a support or pillow in the lower back. To improve posture, always stand and walk tall through the top of your head, to engage all the body's postural muscles.

If you constantly suck in your waist, let go of this unnecessary muscle tension as the pelvic, trunk and upper body postural muscles do their work of holding you upright (and flattening the abdomen).

Case Study

Tina's obstetrician referred her for pelvic floor rehabilitation three weeks after the birth of her first baby. She described a wonderful birth, initially in standing, then in a bath, followed by birth on all fours. Tina stayed constipated for five days after the birth and experienced pain from an internal haemorrhoid. A week after returning home, forceful straining with bowel emptying caused her cervix to prolapse down to the vaginal entrance. Towards the end of each day, she was in pain from both the haemorrhoid and the prolapse, and turned to snack food for comfort.

Tina's depressed mood was evident in her slumped sitting posture. When asked to lift her PF muscles, she pulled her waist back without any pelvic floor lift, which pushed her prolapse down further.

Tina's program started with controlling spinal posture in sitting and standing and she avoided lifting anything heavier than her baby. I asked her to eat more fresh fruit and vegetables, increase her water and fibre intake and adopt the new toilet position (with hand pressure supporting her vagina as the bowel opened), along with regular PF strength exercises.

Tina started PF exercises in sitting then standing, and used the 'knack' to draw up her pelvic floor before lifting.

She was fitted with a vaginal pessary to reposition the cervix and soon reported less pain, and her bowel opened regularly without straining. After months of progressive exercises, Tina was able to lift her baby in his car capsule while controlling her PF muscle lift. She started walking, bike riding and swimming for fitness and weight loss. When time allowed, she enjoyed Fitball and modified one-on-one pilates sessions for ongoing pelvic floor and core strengthening.

Tina and her partner were keen to have a second baby, but she decided to wait another18 months to fully rehabilitate her pelvic floor, abdominal and trunk strength, knowing she also had to lift a heavy toddler while pregnant.

3. Train your PF muscles

It is common knowledge that athletes reach the top of their field through consistent training.

If you are serious about changing pelvic floor problems, make it a habit to exercise these muscles daily. Pelvic floor control comes when you put in the work. I have witnessed some amazing results in my patients over the years. Women who gain complete or significant improvement in pelvic floor control are devoted to their exercise programs. The winners are the women who do not give up, but realise it takes time to train any muscle group. Add PF exercises to daily activities and focus on improved daily habits until they become an everyday routine.

4. Use Orgasm as a PF Workout

The high level of vaginal tensioning and muscle contraction during orgasm is a brilliant pelvic floor workout. As PF muscles strengthen with training, so will orgasm intensity. A stronger pelvic floor means a stronger orgasm - what an incentive to keep exercising! During orgasm, your PF muscle workout is between five to 15 repetitions at 0.8 second intervals.

Case Study

Alice, a 28 year-old florist, described how prolapse, bladder urgency and worsening constipation were affecting her life. She reported poor sensation during intercourse, with less orgasmic intensity. Prior to her daughter's birth six years earlier, she orgasmed quickly with intense contractions. Alice lost confidence sexually after her partner said he could not feel much sensation during intercourse. She had difficulty retaining a tampon (it often slipped out) and sometimes intercourse was painful. Her work involved prolonged standing and lifting heavy buckets filled with water and flowers. Toward the end of the day, Alice experienced vaginal heaviness (prolapse). She had started PF exercises but with no improvement to her symptoms.

Alice initially found it difficult to learn the correct action of lifting her PF muscles, after years of using them in a bearing down action. With instruction and persistence, she learned the correct lifting action, and reported less bladder urgency. Alice learned to open her bowel without straining, and started a regular walking program (not at the same time).

After progressing to strength exercises, Alice reported less prolapse pressure at the end of the day and intercouse was more comfortable. She was able to lift her pelvic floor prior to picking up buckets of flowers to prevent pelvic organ descent.

Her proudest achievement though, was reconnecting with and strenghtening her pelvic floor resulting in heightened sensation with orgasm.

5. Lose Weight

To start losing weight – ditch the latest fad diet to avoid adding unrealistic stress. Successful long-term weight loss consists of making sustainable changes to the type and quantity of food eaten along with regular exercise.

To stay healthy and control weight gain, your body needs fruits, vegetables, lean protein, complex carbohydrates and healthy oil from nuts, fish and avocados. Join a support group or visit a local dietician for a tailored eating plan which becomes a lifelong way of eating. It is all too easy to eat food without thinking of the effect it will have on your body weight. Try relating food choices to your energy levels, moods and hormones. Think positively about what the right food will do for you and make conscious choices to eat what your body needs on a daily basis.

Your brain will lead your food choice, so reprogram it by thinking about the foods your body needs. This shifts your focus away from foods that fertilise fat cells. Continually eating sweet or fatty foods primes brain receptors to demand more of these foods.

Close your eyes and imagine, spread on a table, two to three pieces of fruit and five to seven serves of vegetables, two to three serves of protein, two to three serves of dairy, four to five serves of either whole grain bread, high fibre cereal, nuts, rice, beans or pasta. These foods are recommended on a daily basis to maintain health and prevent weight gain especially when combined with my favourite strategy to control daily intake: serve your meal on a smaller plate. You will eat less yet still see a full plate of food every mealtime. Satisfying the eyes goes a long way to satisfying the appetite!

Combine sensible eating with *some* exercise or physical activity *every day of your life*. Add incidental exercise such as using stairs, walking to the local store or taking children to school. Gardening and dancing through housework to favourite tunes will improve fitness and energy levels.

Keep exercising – find activities you enjoy and it will no longer be a 'chore'.

Damaging Pelvic Floor Habits

1. Heavy Lifting

Pressure increases inside the abdomen with lifting, coughing and excercise are controlled by PF and core muscles. Without a quick, strong PF muscle lift to counter internal pressure, incontinence and prolapse are likely. Figure 6 shows the effect of intra abdominal pressure when the PF muscles are weak or uncoordinated.

A study in Denmark compared assistant nurses with women in the general population. Results showed a significant increased risk of pelvic organ prolapse and lumbar disc herniations in the nursing group, which was attibuted to their occupational heavy lifting. Women working as labourers and factory workers also have a high risk of developing pelvic organ prolapse due to the heavy lifting and prolonged standing.

Early signs of prolapse include poor bladder control, difficult and incomplete bowel emptying, rectal and/or vaginal pain and vaginal heaviness.

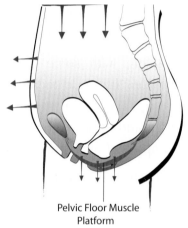

Pelvic Floor Muscle
Platform

When litfting or coughing, depression occurs
if the Pelvic Floor and Transversus are weak
and do not lift with quick strength.

Fig. 6 – Pelvic Floor Depression and Prolapse

2. Excessive Abdominal Training

Sit-ups, curl-ups and double leg lifts have traditionally been recommended for abdominal strengthening. You may be surprised to learn how these exercises affect PF muscles. The sit-up action increases internal abdominal pressure which must be countered by an early, quick, strong pelvic floor lift and hold. If the pelvic floor is weak or slow to respond, it will fail to hold during exercise. Repeating exercises to strengthen the large, powerful abdominal muscles sets the scene for the smaller PF muscles to be overwhelmed and strained.

Weak PF muscles are not the only problem associated with

excessive abdominal training. Some women develop too much PF muscle tone from constantly holding the floor drawn up during exercise sessions. Without periods of relaxation, the PF muscles, over time, become stiff and shortened, losing their ability to relax. Symptoms of increased PF muscle resting tone are urgency, frequency, difficult bladder or bowel emptying, muscular trigger points and painful intercourse.

Sit-ups are not a functional activity; we do not walk around crunching our trunk forwards through the day. We walk, push, lift, carry, sneeze, squat and laugh during a typical day. To cope with these activities, the PF and core muscles benefit from being trained to hold and coordinate with the bracing action of the outer abdominals.

Sit-ups do not shift abdominal fat. A flatter abdomen is achieved through general weight loss combined with inner core muscle exercise targeting the transversus abdominis. This muscle flattens the abdomen and you will soon learn the benefits of keeping it active throughout the day as part of correct posture and PF muscle training.

In Section 3 you will be guided to **find** the PF muscle lift, to coordinate the PF and core muscles and **control** them with specific exercises. Finally you will learn to **train** the pelvic floor and core with the trunk muscles and incorporate this action into your exercise programs.

> *Activating the core by 'pulling the navel back to the spine' is an old and ineffective strategy. The new way is to use a pelvic floor lift to co-tension the deep abdominal muscles.*

Case Study

A friend referred 45 year-old Kate who described bladder urgency and frequency, and a recent bulge at her vaginal entrance. Eight months earlier she commenced a gym program after her DEXA scan showed lumbar osteopenia (early stage osteoporosis). While the gym program was ideal for improving bone density, it was the last straw for her pelvic floor. When I asked Kate to lift her pelvic floor, she strongly tightened her abdominal muscles. This action increased internal abdominal pressure and her floor descended instead of lifting. Starting sit-ups and adding a heavy weights program further increased internal pressure down onto Kate's pelvic floor, leading to vaginal prolapse.

I asked Kate to put her gym membership on hold for six months and replace with walking and swimming. After learning the correct pelvic floor lifting action, she progressed to pelvic floor strength exercises. When Kate returned to the gym, her focus was on combining and training her PF and core strength with a seated program of stretch bands, light weights and Fitball exercises. Her awareness of controlling PF and core muscles during training gave her confidence to continue exercising safely.

> *To reduce injury risk, your pelvic floor should always hold against the exercise load.*

3. Frequent Voiding

Avoid the habit of frequent toilet trips by learning to delay voiding until you have at least 250–300mls in your bladder (a cupful). Aim to empty your bladder no more than five or six times a day and once at night.

Caffeinated drinks and some artificial sweeteners aggravate bladder urgency. If you experience bladder urgency, avoid caffeine – coffee, tea, soft drinks with caffeine and diet colas. Green tea (the early, unfermented stage of black tea) also contains caffeine. Alcohol relaxes bladder control, occasionally leading to unexpected loss of urine with laughing or walking.

There is a lot of truth in the statement that bladder urgency is 'all in your head'. If you feel the urge to void after recently emptying - ignore it. Distract yourself and over-ride the message, allowing the bladder to refill. To gain lasting control over urgency, tighten and lift your PC muscle – the muscle responsible for closing the sphincters at the base of the bladder and urethra; the action you will learn in 'Find It' (page 44). The PC is your body's inbuilt mechanism to control bladder urgency.

To overcome urgency, curl your toes under firmly, tighten the PC muscle and breathe with a relaxed waist until the urge passes. Repeat this action to quieten the bladder rather than giving in to the urge, and start to break free from the tyranny of an urgent bladder.

Document your bladder emptying pattern and volume of urine passed, using the Bladder Chart (page 149). Over a 48 hour period, collect and measure the volume of urine passed and note down the time. Repeat this 48 hour test every month to monitor improvements in bladder control.

Medication may be aggravating bladder frequency, urgency, hesitancy or urinary retention, so ask the pharmacist to supply information sheets regarding prescribed medication and read the side effects section. If side effects include bladder problems, visit your doctor for a medication review.

Regularly drink water throughout the day. Many women with urgency and frequency restrict their fluid intake to control urine loss. Drinking less does not control bladder urgency, and results in fatigue, dehydration and constipation.

Avoid bearing down during voiding; sit tall and relax the abdominal wall to release muscle tension. If the abdomen is held tightly during voiding, the urethral sphincters cannot relax and bearing down is adopted to empty the bladder.

Frequently over riding messages from a full bladder is also risky. When a workplace imposes break times (eg: banks or shops), some women store large urine volumes using PF contractions to over ride bladder emptying signals. Regularly storing volumes over 500ml of urine distends the bladder, reducing its ability to effectively contract while emptying.

> *Avoid frequent hovering above the toilet seat as muscle tension in buttock, pelvic and abdominal muscles makes it difficult for the bladder to fully empty. Use disposable toilet seat liners or antiseptic wipes.*

4. Constantly Drawing in the Waist

The habit of drawing in the waist in to make it appear smaller causes problems for the pelvic floor. Researchers looked at how the PF muscles of continent and incontinent women responded during unexpected loading to their arms. The first muscle response from the continent women was an automatic tightening of their PF muscles (which also activated other core muscles). The incontinent women responded by automatically tightening their waist (external oblique) muscles first with the resultant increase in abdominal pressure exceeding their PF muscle control.

Figure 7 shows the difference between the incontinent woman on the left using her abdominal muscles, compared to the coordinated action of the continent women on the right.

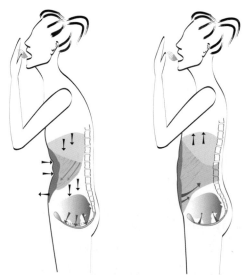

Pelvic Floor lifting activates other core muscles

Fig. 7 – Abdominal Muscle Action in Stress Incontinent and Continent Women

The researchers expected the stress incontinent women would have weaker PF muscles than the continent women. This was not the case, as results showed the PF muscles in the stress incontinent women worked harder than in the continent women, yet they still failed to prevent urine loss.

Sucking in the waist to flatten the abdomen is a habit that contributes to incontinence. You will soon read about the importance of 'letting go' of excessive tension around the waist and rib cage before lifting and strengthening your PF muscles.

5. Running if You Leak

Leaking during running indicates the pelvic floor is not coping with the impact of foot strike plus the load from above of intestines and pelvic organs pushing down. You may feel fine running but cannot see what is happening inside, as supporting tissues stretch to failure point.

Change to low impact exercise incorporating postural control with walking, swimming or bike riding. Focus on learning correct pelvic floor lifting, control and strengthening (or maybe relaxation in some cases). Develop core control with exercises that promote pelvic floor lift and hold while the outer abdominals brace (the normal action with coughing). Start carefully with abdominal strengthening as high level core exercises in a class situation will be too difficult for some women. Relax the pelvic floor between exercises and stop if the muscles become fatigued and fail to hold.

If you decide to return to running, gradually increase the time and intensity of runs over several months, and monitor how your pelvic floor responds to the gradual increases in load and endurance. As you return to leak-free running, continue to balance this activity with ongoing pelvic floor and core exercises.

Case Study

Megan, a 32 year-old chiropractor, sought advice after the birth of her second baby. She was fit and slim, and resumed running 12 weeks post-birth. At six months, she returned to work part-time. She was still breastfeeding and her periods had not returned.

Megan was concerned because she leaked urine after running a few kilometres, but continued despite ongoing loss. The impact loading of running had unmasked her poor pelvic floor control.

She needed much convincing to stop running and start walking instead. With practice, she correctly lifted and strengthened her pelvic floor in conjunction with using vaginal oestrogen pessaries.

After four months of PF muscle strengthening, she was able to run without urine loss, and complemented this with Fitball exercises to develop core strength. Megan was highly motivated to maintain pelvic floor strength exercises so she could continue jogging.

> *Rather than allowing pelvic floor problems stop you from being active, find other suitable, less demanding types of exercise. Inactivity leads to weight gain, muscle weakness and perhaps depression. Abdominal weight gain and weak PF muscles set the scene for future problems.*

Training the Pelvic Floor

3

Preparing for Pelvic Floor Success

Before introducing the three stages of my *Hold It Sister* pelvic floor training program, there are two critical factors to discuss. Please do not rush through this section. Your long-term success with any pelvic floor program relies on a foundation of tall posture, breathing and correct action of the pubococcygeus muscle.

For some women, the posture and breathing come easily; others need to work harder to overcome a lifetime of faulty patterns and habits. It is important to do each of the practical exercises listed below and make any changes needed, before moving to the next stage of the *Hold It Sister* program. Failure to do this is the best way to sabotage your success.

To start preparing for pelvic floor success, sit on a chair facing a mirror and work through the following practical sessions, while watching how your abdominal muscles respond.

1. Posture

PRACTICAL SESSION

Sit and place both hands under your buttocks to find the 'sitting bones'; now slump and roll the weight back onto your sacrum. Feel how slumping shuts down pelvic floor and core postural muscles; they 'let go' (Fig. 8).

Lift up your chest and grow tall through the crown of your head. Feel how this action engages PF and inner core muscles to hold you upright against gravity. If you are tightening waist muscles back, release this extra tension as the core muscles maintain upright posture. You may feel lighter as your postural muscles stiffen around joints to accommodate the load of gravity.

Some women feel uncomfortable letting their waist relax after a lifetime of trying to narrow it! Surprisingly, it is the inner cylinder of core muscles (working with the pelvic floor) that flattens your stomach. To achieve a firmer abdomen, the first step is staying upright in sitting, standing and walking, to keep the PF and core muscles active.

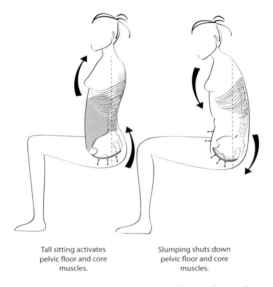

Tall sitting activates
pelvic floor and core
muscles.

Slumping shuts down
pelvic floor and core
muscles.

Fig. 8 – Sitting Posture and the Pelvic Floor

Sitting and standing tall are essential lifetime endurance exercises for the trunk postural muscles. Long hours at the computer, driving or watching television reinforces slumped posture. Tall posture needs frequent practice before it becomes an automatic action. With practice, you will develop the awareness and muscle endurance required to stay tall for longer periods throughout the day. Keeping these muscles active with upright posture has the added benefit of reducing unnecessary wear and tear to the joints during daily activity.

2. Correct breathing

The diaphragm is a musculofibrous partition separating the chest and abdominal cavities. It attaches at the front into the base of the ribs and into the spine via two long tendons. This large muscle performs most of the breathing action. Incorrect patterns of breathing prevent the diaphragm from smoothly moving down and up as you breathe in and out.

The base of the ribs and abdomen should open out as you breathe in, while the shoulders stay relaxed. Holding tension at the waist forces the chest and shoulders to lift up on the in-breath.

Correct Breathing Pattern   Incorrect Breathing Pattern

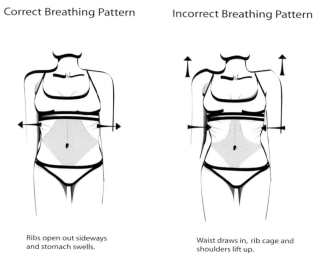

Ribs open out sideways
and stomach swells.

Waist draws in, rib cage and
shoulders lift up.

Fig. 9 – Breathing Patterns

Altered diaphragmatic movement impacts on the pelvic floor as these two muscle partitions have a coordinated pattern of movement. To draw air into the lungs the diaphragm is actively lowered and the pelvic floor slightly descends while maintaining muscle tension and support. On the out-breath, the diaphragm relaxes and recoils upwards to push air from the lungs and the pelvic floor rises with it. Tension in the waist muscles interferes with diaphagmatic descent by preventing the rib cage from widening at the base to allow air into the lower lungs. When the chest wall and waist remain tense, the shoulders are raised to suck air into the lungs. This altered pattern changes the diaphragmatic and pelvic floor contribution to normal breathing.

Slumped posture leaves the diaphragm no room to descend while breathing in, which in turn prevents PF muscles working effectively. In other words, correct breathing relies on correct posture and opening of the base of the ribs.

Watch your chest and ribs in the mirror. Upper chest breathers overuse neck and shoulder muscles to help draw air into their lungs (which contributes to neck and shoulder problems). If your chest and shoulders lift on the in-breath, work through the following steps in the practical session.

PRACTICAL SESSION

Sit in front of a mirror and place a tape measure firmly around the base of your ribs. When you breathe in slowly and deeply, use your side rib expansion to open the tape (see Fig. 10). Repeat 5 times.

If it is difficult to learn a smooth, easy pattern of breathing

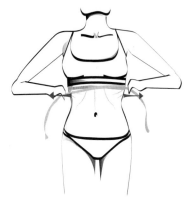

Lower ribs open on the in breath to expand the tape.
Shoulders stay flat.

Fig. 10 - Learning Correct Breathing

while seated, lie on your back with both knees bent. Place both hands on the abdomen, over the base of your ribs, close your eyes and feel what happens under your hands while breathing. Start to gently open your ribs and swell the stomach under your hands as you breathe in, and relax slowly on the out breath.

During breathing the outer abdominal muscles release on the in breath, then the inner abdominal and PF muscles automatically and lightly contract on the out breath. At different times during the day, become aware of your breathing and practice four or five slow, rib-opening breaths. Feel how slow breathing breaks 'guarded' tension around the chest wall and waist.

Breathing is an automatic action normally taken for granted. Being mindful of your breathing is the first step in changing a faulty pattern (perhaps due to a history of asthma, rigid abdominal holding and fear or anxiety states). Yoga stretches and spinal mobilization reduces stiffness in the rib/spinal joints and inter-rib muscles, to allow easier chest expansion.

3. Discovering Down Under

To become more familiar with this amazing part of your body, start by getting to know your pelvic floor from the outside in. Either sit on the edge of a chair, squat, or prop up with pillows on your bed with a hand mirror angled to view your pelvic floor.

Start by feeling the mons pubis (covered by pubic hair) and the pubic bone underneath. Move down to the clitoris and draw back the covering hood to expose the sensitive tip or glans. The thicker, outer labia (majora) are covered with hair; parting the inner labia (minora) reveals the urethral and vaginal openings. The vestibule is the area surrounding the vaginal opening and the area between the vagina and anus is the perineum.

Vulva is the name given to the area around the vaginal opening; the labia minora and majora and the clitoris. Images from the powerful fashion and pornographic industries may lead women to question their individual and unique body shapes. Women have marked variations between feet, breasts, fingers, legs and just about every anatomical area, and it is normal for clitoral and labial sizes to range from smaller to larger and vary in colour. Fig. 11 will help you find your way around.

Superficial muscles (ischiocavernosus, bulbocavernosus) close the vaginal opening. The perineum is supported and strengthened by the transverse perineal muscle that connects to the deeper PF muscles (levator ani) which lift internally to close sphincters and support organs.

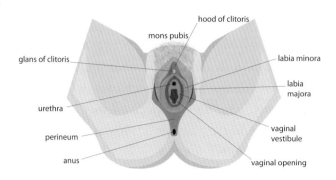

Fig. 11 - The Pelvic Floor External View

An effective PF muscle action involves closing the vagina, lifting up internally to raise the pelvic floor and switch on the other core muscles.

Finding Your PC Muscle Action

These five practical tips are ways to learn the effective lifting action by initially observing and feeling the correct action of pubococcygeus (PC), an important PF muscle involved in bladder continence and sexual response. The PC has a right and left sided attachment to the back of the pubic bone, and along with the puborectalis muscle (which loops around the anal sphincter) joins into the coccyx and lower sacrum. Together these muscles compress the anal, vaginal and urethral openings, with internal lifting.

The PC lift is felt at the front of the pelvic floor, whereas the anal sphincter lift (puborectalis) is felt at the back of the pelvic floor. Initially, you will learn to identify your PC muscle before training it to lift and strengthen with all the PF muscles.

Find which of the following actions helps you recognise the internal lifting action of your PC muscle. I have included a training action after each item to improve awareness of this muscle in action. Release any embarrassment with self-examination: instead use this as a chance to become more familiar with how your pelvic floor works. These exercise skills are essential for pregnant and postpartum strengthening but ideally are adopted for every day PF muscle control throughout life.

1. Mirror, Mirror

Sit on the edge of a chair and angle a mirror to view your pelvic floor. Open your legs and part the labial lips. Observe what happens when you lift your PC (while breathing out), as though trying to stop the flow of urine. You should see closing and a slight lift of the urethral and vaginal openings. The anal sphincter draws in but focus the lift to the front of the pelvic floor with thighs, buttocks and waist relaxed.

Repeat, and focus on a slow closing and lifting of the urethral and vaginal openings. Observe the floor relaxation when letting go of the lift.

Now watch what happens to your pelvic floor duing a strong cough. If it bulges down, the PC and other muscles are either weak or slow to respond. This may also happen during activity or exercise when it should tighten and lift. Failing to correct this faulty pattern of pelvic floor descent will lead to incontinence and pelvic organ prolapse. If the floor 'holds' when coughing, your PF muscles tightened at the right time.

Action: Become aware of tightening and lifting the pelvic floor before you cough or lift. Learn the PC lift and repeat this action when standing, walking, coughing and lifting. While this may be initially difficult, keep practicing until it becomes a more familiar action.

2. Tampon Tug

Wash your hands before swelling a tampon with warm water, and inserting vaginally. Try to keep the tampon in place while pulling slowly on the string. If the tampon holds and you need to pull more firmly, this shows your PC is tightening. If the tampon pulls out easily, then the muscle lacks effective strength.

Action: Reinsert the tampon, gently pull on the string and tighten and lift vaginally to hold the tampon in place for five seconds. Relax and repeat 5 to 8 times. Remove and discard tampons after use.

3. Hold It Sister

This activity is not an exercise, but a way to help identify the sensation of using your PC muscle. Try to stop the flow of urine during bladder emptying but only try this occasionally, as your bladder should empty in a continuous stream.

Action: Try this action no more than once a week, as a gauge of muscular control.

4. Feel Your PC Action

Insert your index and middle fingers about an inch into your vagina. Repeat the PC lift to feel squeezing and drawing-up around your fingers; this is the correct action of the muscle.

A healthy muscle feels full and firm around the fingers and a weak muscle feels soft with less response. A variation in muscle size and squeeze pressure between right and left sides may be noted. If nothing happens or the lift is minimal, the muscle is either weak or damaged, or you don't understand the lifting action of the muscle.

If inserting fingers is difficult or painful, this indicates PF muscle tightness or a type of vulval pain syndrome.

Action: If muscle tightening is absent or the insertion is painful, consult a gynaecologist to rule out any pathology or disease and visit a physiotherapist who specialises in treating PF muscles, to discuss your findings.

5. The Right Vibe

Vibration gives increased sensory input to muscles. Many women have discovered the benefits of using a vibrator to reach orgasm, but less known is that vibration increases a muscle's ability to contract, improving its strength.

If you use a vibrator, insert it vaginally (with a little lubricant), and tighten your PC around the vibrator. A definite closing and squeezing action around the vibrator should be felt.

Action: Insert the vibrator and repeat PC tightening and relaxation, holding for 5 to 10 seconds, then relax before repeating. If your PC fatigues (the tightening action becomes difficult), take a break to let your muscles relax.

The purpose of these activities is to learn the local action of the PC muscle in your pelvic floor. This is only the beginning of developing effective pelvic floor control. Soon you will use the PC action in different exercise combinations. Practising the following exercises builds control and strength in your pelvic floor during daily activity, lifting and exercising.

What are Kegel Exercises?

'Kegels' is the American term used for the PF exercises developed by Dr Arnold Kegel. In 1948 he advised, 'It is a good idea in all cases that have been operated on for prolapse of the vagina vault or uterus, or in every postpartum woman to teach them how to contract the vaginal musculature and let them use this as a prophylactic measure.'

Kegels have become one of the most misunderstood exercises. Many of my clients had done 'Kegels' for years but remained incontinent or unable to control prolapse. 'Kegels' on their own, even if done well, do not develop the integrated PF and core muscle activity identified as critical in the newer research on which *Hold It Sister* is based.

Find It. Control It. Train It.

With a clearer understanding of posture and breathing, we now move on to the *Hold It Sister* pelvic floor training program.

There are three stages – beginning with finding the correct muscle action, then strengthening the PF muscles and finally training the PF muscles to cope with heavier or unexpected loading.

Avoid rushing the early 'Find It' stage; take time to learn the correct PC action before progressing to the 'Control It' phase. Be confident you have mastered the first stage before moving on to ensure the best possible long term outcome.

Find It

PRACTICAL SESSION

- Sit tall and lean forwards to rest forearms on your legs, with bottom well out behind in the chair. If you normally hold your waist drawn back, practice abdominal wall release by placing a hand over your stomach and feeling the softening release of muscle tension.
- Breathe in slowly and deeply, expanding the base of your ribs and breathe out continuously through pursed lips.
- On the next long out breath, imagine slowly drawing a tampon back in vaginally. This is a slow, gentle lifting movement, starting from underneath the body, to feel the PC action without other muscles jumping in first. Hold this tension and breath to avoid breath holding.
- Feel how your urethra and vagina close and lift slightly in an upward direction.
- If this PF muscle action is difficult to feel in sitting, try side lying for easier stomach relaxation. Move back to sitting when you feel confident the action is correct.

If you struggle to identify the muscle action, try a different mental cue. Imagine a sharp needle coming towards your urethra and vagina. Slowly close your urethra and vagina and lift up internally away from the imaginary needle as you breathe out continuously through pursed lips.

If done correctly, a gentle urethral and vaginal lifting is felt along with firmness at your bikini line and maybe lower back. This second sensation is transversus abdominis and deep spinal postural muscles working with the PF muscles. This exercise teaches you three things; firstly how to lead the PF lift action with the PC muscle, secondly how subtle the PC action is, and finally how the PC muscle brings in the other core muscles.

Relax and start again until you feel the gentle tension between your pelvic floor and deep core muscles. Many of my clients say they hardly feel anything and this is normal as the PC action is slow with gentle lifting in the early learning stage. The sensation is different from what you feel when tightening a strength muscle. It is the difference between the effort of lightly squeezing the tip of the index finger and thumb together compared with the effort of making a strong fist.

Some women find their PC muscle 'flickers' initially. This gradually becomes a sustained muscle hold as they continue the action of slowly tightening and relaxing the PC muscle.

Hold for five to ten seconds as you breathe. Do five to eight repetitions, being sure to relax the floor after each one. Repeat this at least four times every day.

> *If your PF muscles let go while breathing, you are probably using the outer tummy muscles first, instead of the gentler PF muscles. Relax and try again more slowly.*

Expect to find PF exercises more difficult to learn in standing, as the stronger outer abdominal muscles are primed to switch on early in some women. Try leaning forwards onto a bench, soften both knees and tilt your bottom upwards (to increase the arch in your lower back) and completely relax your abdominal wall. Some women find it easier to feel the vaginal lift in this position.

Other women try to flatten their stomach by breathing in and pulling their waist back strongly instead of 'growing tall' and using pelvic floor lifting with the associated deep abdominal tensioning, to find stomach control. Working through these exercises will encourage you to slow down and become aware of tension unconsciously held around the waist and ribs. This awareness is the key to establishing a more effective brain and pelvic floor connection.

BE PATIENT with yourself in this learning stage and let go of frustration, as it takes time to re-program a new muscle action. Initially your brain may not know what you are trying to do, as it struggles to learn and recognise the gentle closing, lifting action of the PC muscle. Close your eyes, and go back to waist softening with slower basal rib breathing before trying again.

The reason for breaking down the steps in learning the correct PC lift is to identify what the action feels like. With regular practice, it may become automatic. Your anal sphincter muscle (puborectalis) should close and lift with the PC muscle, to draw the entire floor upwards. In this early stage, focus the action to the front of your floor. Most women find they can tighten and lift their anal sphincter, but are not able to draw up the PC (which should happen first). The next section involves pelvic floor strength exercises with the anal sphincter lift. Only move to the next exercise stage when you are confident in your ability to lift the PC first. If you cannot lift your PC after re-practicing all the earlier steps, seek assistance from a women's health physiotherapist.

Substitution

When PF muscles are damaged, weak or uncoordinated, outer abdominal, buttock and back muscles may substitute for the gentle PF and inner core muscles. Fig. 12 shows the outer abdominal muscle substitution that increases internal abdominal pressure.

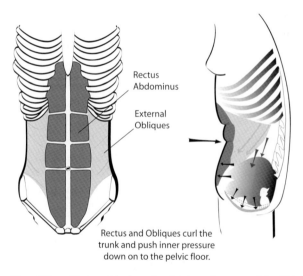

Rectus
Abdominus

External
Obliques

Rectus and Obliques curl the
trunk and push inner pressure
down on to the pelvic floor.

Fig. 12 – Outer Abdominal Muscles used in Waist
Tensioning

Continuing to tighten or strengthen the upper abdominals contributes to PF dysfunction. When supporting ligaments stretch, they fail to support the bladder, vagina, uterus and bowel, allowing the pelvic organs to sag down into the vaginal walls (prolapse).

Figure 4, on page 7, shows the correct muscle action to use before coughing, picking up a toddler or turning a heavy mattress on your bed. Learn and repeat the action until it becomes automatic in your body to help protect your spine from injury, to maintain continence and prevent prolapse.

Retraining May Be Difficult for Some

Retraining the brain to reprogram a complex sequence of muscle actions is always difficult. In the early stages of learning, the brain prefers the old pattern, especially when under stress or not concentrating. Overcoming the old pattern and replacing it with a new pattern involves focused practice. Hundreds of *correct* repetitions are needed to avoid any lapse into the old pattern. This can take weeks or months.

Women using the outer abdominal tightening pattern will have the most difficulty learning the new action. Be patient until you are confidently lifting the PC from underneath first.

Many women use too much effort when learning PF exercises, and tighten waist, leg and buttock muscles, which reinforces an incorrect action.

Obviously, not all women hold their waist tightly drawn back. A slack, protruding abdomen also indicates the PF and core muscles are not working to flatten the abdomen and support the internal pelvic organs.

Forget about strength in the early FIND IT stage. It is difficult to find the inner muscles if using more than a slow, gentle lifting action. *This stage of learning has nothing to do with strength; it is about locating and coordinating the muscles in a gentle manner, so your brain learns the correct sensation without stronger muscles dominating the action.*

> **Relax and slow down to find the softer, lifting action of your PC muscle.**

Don't even try to strengthen until you can lift the PF muscles without the stronger muscles jumping in first. When you are confidently lifting the PC first from underneath your body, start internally lifting and squeezing the muscles more firmly.

The next stage is improving STRENGTH with five to six months of regular PF exercises.

Control It

I hope you are gaining a new respect for your PC. It is a remarkable muscle working across the whole spectrum of activity, from slow to fast, from gentle to strong and deserves daily attention.

Pelvic floor muscles experience three levels of strength and endurance.

- The PF muscles stay constantly switched on at a low level during the day when you are sitting or walking tall. This is LOW LEVEL ENDURANCE.

- The PF muscles combine strength and endurance for sustained load activities — for example: uphill walking or carrying a child. This is STRENGTH ENDURANCE.

- The PF muscles react rapidly with any sudden, unexpected loading — for example: when you sneeze or trip. This is QUICK STRENGTH.

As PF muscles have multiple actions, three separate training exercises are required to prepare your muscles for different daily activities.

Exercise 1: Endurance

Every morning, start with the gentle PC lifting exercise to reinforce the correct lifting action and then advance the action with a little more endurance training.

While sitting or standing, grow tall and relax waist tightness. Breathe out, slowly lift the PC and hold for 10-30 seconds, while breathing. Repeat this light lifting action at different times during the day.

Activity: When you sit or walk, grow tall through the crown of your head and feel this lengthening automatically switch on the PC and deep abdominal (core) tension. Improving postural control is the easiest and most effective way to keep the low-level endurance of your PC active.

Exercise 2: Strength

Start this exercise in sitting, with a relaxed waist. Breathing out, lift your PC and continue drawing up higher and higher vaginally, along with squeezing and lifting your anal sphincter. Hold and breathe for 10 seconds. Relax completely for 5 to 10 seconds and repeat 5 to 8 times.

Stay focused on deep internal vaginal lifting and with the stronger lift, feel all the abdominal muscles working together.

If dizziness is felt, too much effort is being used. Progress the exercise to standing. Place both hands on a table, lean forwards and stick your bottom out behind. Tilt your bottom up lengthen through your crown, relax the waist and soften your knees. This position helps you isolate and start the lift from the front of the pelvic floor. Also try this exercise kneeling on hands and knees with forehead resting on forearms or sitting on the floor in an open, crossed-legged pose.

Activity: Pelvic floor descent with exercise weakens internal organ supports. A good test of pelvic floor functional strength is holding the pelvic floor lift while standing from a squat. Train your PF muscles to lift before and hold during the movement as squatting is an everyday action.

Exercise 3: Quick Strength

To ensure your pelvic floor reacts quickly when coughing, sneezing or jumping, practice this third exercise.

In sitting, quickly and strongly lift your pelvic floor, hold for 2-3 seconds, then relax completely. Do 8-10 of these quick, strong internal lifts, and rest when the muscles fatigue.

Repeat quick lifts to train an early pelvic floor response to sudden movement. Try quick PF lifting and holding with simulated coughing, first in tall sitting, then in standing.

How Much is Enough?

For the three exercises (endurance, strength and quick strength) to be effective, follow a training routine.

- Start by repeating each of the three exercises three times per day, starting with five and increasing to 10 repetitions per session. Add a second set of each exercise (after a 60 second rest) in 4-6 weeks time.

- To gain more benefit from the strength exercises, practice them in different positions: sitting, kneeling on all fours (head down), open leg sitting then progress to leaning forward while standing, upright standing, and standing up from squatting.

- Using a vibrator or biofeedback probe provides a resistance to the internal squeezing, lifting action.

- Continue the three exercises to ensure all three modes of pelvic floor action are developed.

- PF muscle relaxation between contractions prevents hyperactivity and allows for more effective strengthening.

- If PF muscles are hyperactive, continue only with the first exercise (low level endurance) and seek the advice of a women's health physiotherapist.

Activity: Repeat these exercises daily for 30 days to ensure they become part of your health routine. Stick a calendar on your bathroom mirror or wall and mark off each day of practice. On completion of day 30, you are officially a pelvic floor athlete!

Pelvic floor muscle strengthening takes around 5 to 6 months for most women. After this initial training period continue with one set of exercises most days of the week to maintain pelvic muscle strength.

The Protective Bracing Pattern

Maybe you are a regular at the gym, returning to exercise after giving birth or have decided to lose weight and tone up. Great planning goes into organising exercise clothes, the best sports shoes and regular times to exercise. Probably the last thing considered is how exercise could affect your pelvic floor.

If occasional leaks have you avoiding certain exercises or activities, learning to recruit the pelvic floor and all the abdominal muscles *together* will improve pelvic floor control during exercise.

The **Protective Bracing Pattern (PBP)** provides this final link.

PRACTICAL SESSION

The final exercise starts with identifying what happens to your pelvic floor *and* abdominal muscles during coughing.

Sit upright with waist relaxed; push your hands *firmly* into the sides of your waist. Cough *strongly* and feel the waist widen out sideways under your hands. Now repeat the same action and note what your pelvic floor does during the cough.

If your pelvic floor lifts and holds with coughing then the PF and core muscles automatically tightened together, as the outer abdominal muscles braced.

This action of pelvic floor lifting, with the front abdomen flattening and side waist widening, is your body's protective bracing pattern (PBP).

If the waist narrows under the hands, the abdomen bulges to the front or your pelvic floor pushes down, then the floor is not coordinating with other core and abdominal muscles.

Retraining the pelvic floor to lift with abdominal muscle contraction is now a priority. Retry the 'cough test' focusing on the pelvic floor lift before the cough. If you are not confident, return to learning the gentle pelvic floor and deep core action, as well as the quick strength exercise, for rapid pelvic floor lifting with simulated coughing.

The final step to total PF coordination is learning the PBP as an exercise, as a strong, coordinated PBP protects the bladder against leaking, prevents prolapse and supports the spine during exercise or lifting. Learning this action provides an understanding of the control needed with exercise, rather than pushing your body to perform difficult tasks. If the pelvic floor descends or the abdomen bulges with exercise, stop the activity and select an easier option.

Activity: Sit upright and push both hands firmly into the sides of your waist. Make a strong 'hissing' sound and feel the waist widen out into your hands.

Watch in the mirror to avoid bending forward at the waist. Relax, repeat this action (stay tall), lift the pelvic floor first and feel the waist widen as you hiss.

When the pelvic floor lifts and holds with waist widening, you have the correct PBP. Always lift from the pelvic floor first when repeating this exercise. Notice the difference between the abdomen flattening and widening at the side waist compared to the action of sucking in the navel and crunching forward to flatten the abdomen.

Hold the PBP for 5 to 10 seconds; relax and repeat 5 to 10 times. Progress this same action to standing. Practice the PBP daily to strengthen this pattern and start integrating the action with exercise and daily activity.

Train It

Once you have mastered the pelvic floor lift and integrated the PBP, start training your pelvic floor as part of a total body program.

The following pages show examples of exercises using various positions, apparatus and movements which will train all postural muscles, leading with the pelvic floor.

Start the exercises at a slow even pace, and concentrate on correct posture to maintain the pelvic floor action throughout the whole exercise. If you cannot maintain the PF lift or the load or speed of movement is too much, back off a little and work on control.

As your floor coordinates and strengthens, increase the level of resistance of bands or weights, increase the speed of the movements or add to the complexity by standing on a stability disc.

Relax PF muscles between exercises, re-engaging them before you repeat the movement.

Start by practicing the first five exercises 2-3 times a week. If you are feeling comfortable and confident add another exercise each week.

If pregnant, avoid lying on your back to exercise after week 20. Focus instead on the sitting and standing exercises, engaging the PBP before the exercise.

Exercise 1

Hip Bridge

Breathe out, lift the PF muscles and push through your heels to lift hips off the floor. Hold and breathe for 10 seconds. Lower slowly with control and repeat 5-10 times.

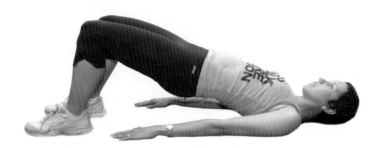

Progress difficulty by slowly raising and lowering both arms during the 10 second hold phase. Keep hips lifted.

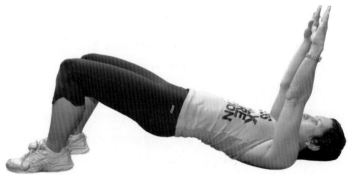

Exercise 2

Arm - Leg Extension

Start on hands and knees and extend one arm and opposite leg. Grow tall through the supporting hip, maintaining good balance and control. Hold and breathe for 10 seconds. Repeat 5 holds then change sides.

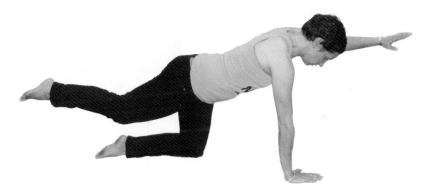

Progress difficulty by maintaining a straight spine as you bring the opposite knee and elbow toward each other, then stretch long again during the ten-second hold phase.

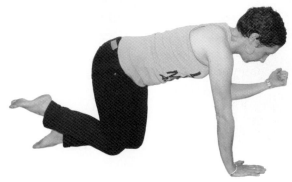

Exercise 3

Sitting Control

• *Sit on the ball in front of a mirror.*

• *Grow tall through your crown.*

• *Lift one foot off the floor.*

• *Hold and breathe for 5-10 seconds.*

• *Alternate left and right foot lifts for 5-10 repetitions.*

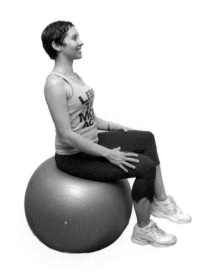

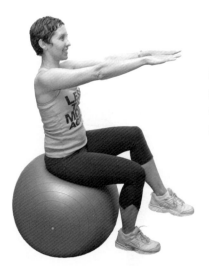

Progress by adding slow double or alternate arm lifts while staying balanced during the 10 second hold phase.

Exercise 4

One Leg Balance.

Stand on one leg and:

• Grow tall through the crown of your head.

• Stay balanced as you raise the other leg to 90° at the hip.

• Lengthen up through the supporting hip and leg.

• Hold and breathe for 10 seconds. Repeat 5 times each leg.

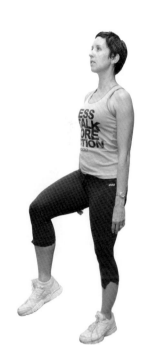

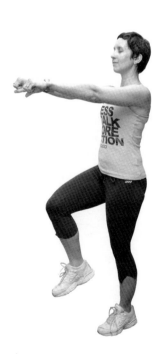

Progress by adding double or alternate arm lifts during the balance phase; stay tall and breathe.

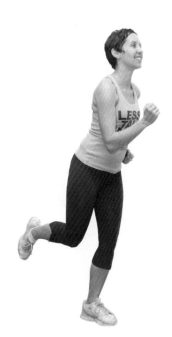

Exercise 5

Stationary Running

In a one-leg balance stance, move your free leg in a forward/backward running action, keeping arms tucked against the body. Only the raised leg moves.

Movement should be slow and controlled, concentrating on balance and smoothness. Stay tall as you move and keep the supporting leg slightly bent.

Once confident with the leg action, progress by using arms in a running crossover action: right leg forward with left arm forward for 30-60 seconds

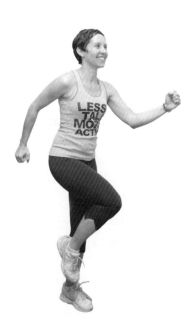

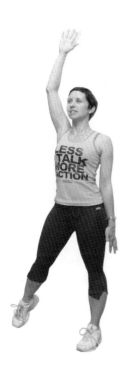

Exercise 6

Overhead Reach with Leg Lift

Stand with weight on one leg with the other leg extended to the side, just touching the floor for balance. Raise the arm on that side overhead.

Grow tall through the crown, raise your knee up to the side and bring your elbow down toward it. Repeat slowly 10 times before changing sides.

Stay tall on the supporting leg as you bring the elbow downwards.

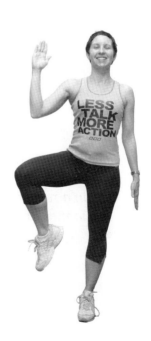

Exercise 7

Wall Squat

• *Place the ball behind your lower back against the wall.*

• *Place feet forward and apart.*

• *Keep pressure on the ball as you squat down, letting the ball roll down the wall.*

• *Push back up through your heels while growing tall through your crown.*

• *Repeat ten times.*

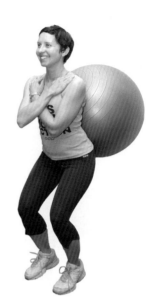

Exercise 8

Chair Squat

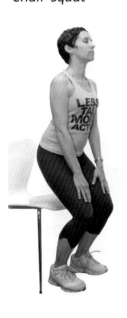

• *Place a chair behind your legs (no wheels).*

• *Stay tall as you SLOWLY control the squat down to touch the chair.*

• *Initially you may need to sit before returning to standing.*

• *Progress to 'touch and slowly lift' as you reach the chair.*

• *Breathe out as you push up through your heels on each of the ten repetitions.*

Exercise 9

Seated Row

Use a lighter band initially.

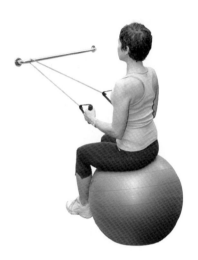

- Sit on a ball or chair.

- Face toward the anchor point of the band.

- Stay tall as you breathe out, lift pelvic floor and slowly pull elbows back.

- Do 5-10 slow repetitions.

Exercise 10

Seated Shoulder Punch

- Sit on a ball or chair.

- Face away from band anchor point.

- Stay tall and lift pelvic floor and slowly punch one arm forwards.

- Repeat 5-10 times with each arm.

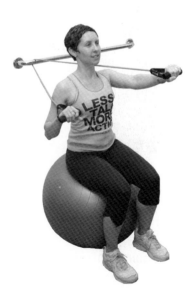

Exercise 11

Standing Arm Draw

For all three exercises:

- *'Retain 'soft' knees. lift the pelvic floor as you breathe out and pull the band in a slow, smooth action.*

- *If you cannot hold your PF lift and breathe, the resistance is too strong; use a lighter band.*

- *Repeat 5-10 times*

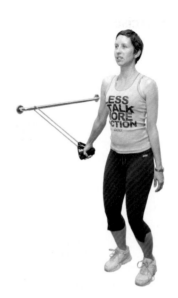

Standing Arm Punch

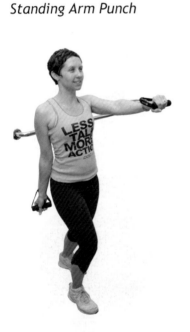

Standing Biceps Curl

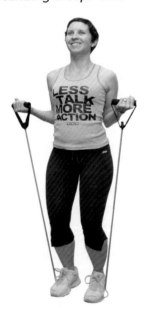

Exercise 12

Balance, Lean, Pick Up

This is a more advanced postpartum exercise - not a pregnancy exercise.

This exercise involves controlling the pelvic floor, core and balance during the action of picking up a small object from the floor while standing on one leg, for 5 repetitions.

If getting to the floor is too challenging, start by placing the object on a chair or coffee table. As your control improves, place the object on progressively lower surfaces.

This exercise requires floor and core activation throughout the bend and pick up movement. Relax when you return to upright stance.

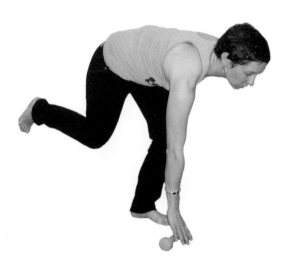

Activity and the Pelvic Floor

4

Sport and The Pelvic Floor

High rates of stress and urge incontinence have been reported in elite female athletes, particularly in running, jumping and landing sports. Researchers report rates of stress incontinence of up to 52 per cent in some sports (varies between sports). Athletes with an eating disorder showed significantly higher rates of incontinence than athletes with normal eating patterns. Competitive elite trampolinists demonstrate high rates of stress incontinence while training, which persists when they leave the sport. Many athletes accept urine loss as part of their sport, using frequent bladder emptying, limited water intake and protective pads to manage the problem.

Physiotherapists working with sporting teams include exercise programs to improve pelvic and lumbar stability as an injury reduction strategy. Including specific PF exercises as part of the training schedule reduces the risk of incontinence in female athletes, along with the increased risk of prolapse and sexual dysfunction later in life.

Women competing in recreational sport experience less urine loss with low impact sports (golf), compared to those involved in running and jumping sports (basketball). Urine loss is often a factor in a woman's decision to give up sport, however avoiding activity leads to loss of strength and muscle mass. Staying active is achievable with continence guards, PF muscle strength programs and switching to a lower impact activity.

Gym and The Pelvic Floor

Throughout history women remained active with walking, gardening, riding, hiking, archery, rowing, tennis, dancing and golf. Daily tasks also provided activity as they played with children, carried loads, climbed stairs, and worked in their homes and gardens.

The growth of fitness centers over the last two decades have many positives as they promote structured exercises for our sedentary society, replacing the incidental exercise previously part of normal work and life activities. Various structured classes promote fitness with spinning, boxing, boot camp, and heavy weights classes. These programs are proving too challenging for some women's level of PF control and contributing to their incontinence and prolapse.

For many gym members, the focus is on exercise classes, individual cardio and strength exercise and personal training sessions. The emphasis is on counting repetitions or minutes, rather than awareness of core control. When the pelvic floor lacks the strength to cope with high demand exercise routines, pelvic supporting structures and muscular control is challenged. Pregnant, postpartum, peri and post menopausal and senior women are at risk of aggravating or causing bladder urgency, incontinence and pelvic organ prolapse with over challenging exercise routines.

When the focus is on sustained or intense PF muscle tensioning, some women are at risk of developing too much tension in the PF muscles. Activities such as advanced core exercises, traditional abdominal classes, prolonged cycling classes or running, do not allow time for muscle relaxation. Without relaxation breaks, PF muscles adapt by developing a higher muscle resting tone, resulting in muscle stiffness, incoordination and pain, along with poor bladder and bowel control.

Women's pelvic health will benefit when specific pelvic function related questions become part of standard exercise assessment forms. Using inadequate pre-participation screening questionnaires, which do not identify information regarding a client's pelvic function and control, exposes women to inappropriate training. Sporting coaches and fitness professionals have a duty of care to women in this regard.

The following Pelvic Health Screening Questions allow the coach or trainer to identify women with, or at risk of developing pelvic floor dysfunction.

Pelvic Health Screening Questions to include in the initial pre-exercise screening form:

- Do you lose urine when you sneeze or run?
- Does bladder urgency cause urine loss?
- Are you currently pregnant?
- Do you have children?
- Mode of birth?
- Any abdominal muscle separation?
- Any recent or chronic low back or pelvic joint pain?
- Any pelvic or spinal surgery?
- Does you mother have a prolapse?
- Any concerns with bowel control?
- Do you regularly exercise PF muscles?

When the answers to the above questions identify at risk women, their exercise program is designed around pelvic control with low impact activities, postural exercises, and seated light strength work. Understanding pelvic floor limitations will empower women to recognise and speak up when the program is too demanding, and encourage them to stay active with appropriate activity throughout life.

Testing to Identify Pelvic and Core Muscle Control:

Try the following activities to help identify your level of pelvic and core muscle control before starting a new exercise program.

- Lie on your back with legs straight and lift one leg a few inches off the floor. If the abdomen bulges upward and the pelvic floor descends, the PF and core muscles are not working to stabilise the pelvis. The curve in the lower back should not flatten during this test. Normally the abdomen firms and flattens with pelvic floor lifting, in response to leg lifting. When one leg feels heavier to lift, specific pelvic muscle and joint imbalances are the likely cause.

- Stand in front of a long mirror and observe your abdomen in the mirror to see what happens when you lift the PF muscles. If you breathed in and tightened back at the waist, or tucked the buttocks under, this indicates the strong upper abdominal and buttock muscles are leading the action. The normal response to a PF muscle lift is a slow lower abdominal firming and navel flattening, with no spinal flattening.

- Again look in the mirror and observe what happens as

you take in a deep breath. If the shoulders lifted with activity in the neck muscles, this indicates an upper chest-breathing pattern with restriction at the base of the ribs. The normal response to deep breathing is sideways expansion of the base of the ribs with little shoulder elevation.

Identifying a faulty action in any of the three tests indicates the need to train the coordination of pelvic floor, core and abdominal muscles with basal rib expansion breathing.

> *Prior to a gym program, develop PF and deep abdominal muscle control before adding challenging exercises.*

Exercise Guidelines For At Risk Clients

1. Avoid over challenging exercise

The pelvic floor is a small muscle group that fatigues with prolonged exercise, and may be overwhelmed with heavy lifting, or exercise focusing on upper abdominal strengthening.

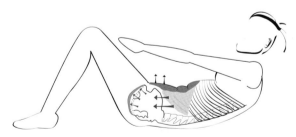

Repeated sit-ups can cause urgency,
urge incontinence and prolapse.

Fig. 13 - Effect of over challenging abdominal
exercises on the pelvic floor

Build strength from the inside out with PF exercises to train pelvic control during exercise. Avoid abdominal exercises that only focus on isolating the abdominal wall muscles. Engage the PBP (p.53) to contract all abdominals during exercise .

2. Focus on core control during exercise

Maintain a tall body posture during exercise to switch on the stabilizing core muscles. Stop the exercise if pelvic muscle control 'lets go', and reduce the exercise intensity or load. For example, if you are working out on a leg extension machine, stay tall as you raise and lower the weight. If you are not able to hold a tall, strong posture, the load is too high for your core control. While your legs may be strong, the core is not providing the pelvic and spinal stability needed to prevent injury.

3. Build in relaxation times

If the pelvic floor fatigues part way through a workout, it lacks endurance and is prone to damage. Repeated fast or high load work may cause loss of core control and substitution of other abdominal muscle strategies to provide trunk stability. Sustained rises in intra abdominal pressure or even one sudden, heavy episode may result in pelvic floor damage in some women.

Alternatively, prolonged vigorous exercise with continued PF muscle contraction results in increased muscle tone in some women. The pelvic floor, like any skeletal muscle, must relax or 'let go' of tension between exercises to prevent hyperactivity. Ensure training activities have opportunities for recovery to reduce fatigue and over activity.

4. Choose suitable exercise

When the pelvic health screening questions and pelvic/core muscle control tests reveal weak or uncoordinated muscles, follow the recommended exercise guidelines:

- Pool exercise.
- Seated bike work.
- Treadmill-keep flat and stay tall while walking.
- Tai chi.
- Seated ball exercises.
- Seated stretch band exercises.
- Hip bridging (on back).
- Opposite arm/leg extensions in four point kneeling.
- Wall squats using a ball behind.
- Basic pilates and reformer exercises.
- Balance activities.
- Cool down with muscle stretches.

Work through these activities for 4 to 6 weeks before:

- Increased repetitions.
- Increased sets.
- Increased band resistance.
- Increased cardio time.

In summary:

- Take the pelvic and core muscle control tests before starting an exercise program to gauge your level of control.
- Control posture throughout the activity to keep postural muscles engaged.

- Lift the pelvic floor as you breathe out on the resisted phase of the exercise, to engage postural muscles.
- Build in rest phases during an exercise session for pelvic floor recovery.
- Urgency, urine loss, pelvic pain or heaviness after exercise, indicates the program (or part of it) is too challenging for pelvic floor control.
- Stay active throughout life with exercise to suit your pelvic floor and core level of control.

Pregnancy, Birth and Postpartum

5

Pregnancy and the Pelvic Floor

While many women sail through pregnancy, others experience aches and pains as their body is transformed. The body has nine months to adapt, and during the later months changes in weight distribution stress the pelvis, spine and pelvic floor. Common pelvic/abdominal conditions include separation of the outer abdominal muscles, sharp abdominal twinges, pelvic girdle pain, low back pain, leg or vulvar varicose veins, constipation and haemorrhoids. This section provides information on how to alleviate and manage conditions affecting the pelvis, abdomen, spine and pelvic floor to improve the pregnancy and birth experience.

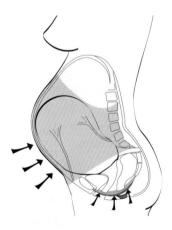

This muscular corset supports the
growing uterus to prevent pain in the
spine, sacroiliac joints and groin.

Fig. 14– Pelvic Floor and Transversus
Provide Support for the Pregnant Uterus

Bladder Control

Pregnancy may be the first time bladder leakage is experienced. The sphincter muscles controlling the 'holding in' of urine are softened by pregnancy hormones (progesterone and relaxin), reducing their firm closure. In early pregnancy these normal hormonal changes plus increased blood flow to the kidneys cause bladder frequency and increased urine production. Some mothers are prone to urinary tract infections in the early stages of pregnancy, while later, toilet trips are more frequent due to uterine pressure on the bladder.

The bladder is pushed forward by the uterus, changing the angle at the bladder neck needed for closure and continence, so leaking may occur. To reduce the likelihood of bladder leaks, start PF exercises during pregnancy and continue after baby is born. Research findings reinforce the importance of controlling leaking during pregnancy.

- The weight of the uterus can weaken and strain the pelvic floor. Studies show regular PF exercises during pregnancy decrease postpartum urinary incontinence.
- Bladder leaking before or during pregnancy, increases the risk of being incontinent after baby is born.
- Weight gain during pregnancy is not associated with increased urinary incontinence, however failure to lose weight gained during pregnancy six months postpartum IS associated with incontinence.
- Results from one study show intensive PF muscle training during pregnancy seems to facilitate labour, and could prevent a prolonged second stage.

Poor bladder control is common immediately after vaginal

and caesarean births and, for the majority of women, this weakness responds well to a committed PF exercise routine.

Such findings underline the need for regular PF exercises to control bladder function during pregnancy. To control bladder urgency, tighten the PC muscle, curl toes under and breathe slowly for 10 seconds or until the sensation fades. Do not restrict fluid intake because of urine loss.

Frequent toilet trips are normal during pregnancy. Before pregnancy the bladder empties five or six times a day and once at night. Increased frequency may also be due to a urinary tract infection (UTI) with associated urethral burning, back pain, nausea or vomiting. Self management includes increased water intake, use of urinary alkalysers and avoiding caffeine. If symptoms persist for 24 hours or become severe, visit your doctor immediately. Untreated UTIs can lead to more serious kidney infection.

Pelvic Girdle Pain

The pelvic girdle transmits weight between the upper and lower body and maintains dynamic stability by balanced posture and synergistic muscle action. Pregnancy weight gains, centre of gravity changes, strenuous work, previous injury, increased BMI, hormones, daily postures, exercise habits, position of baby (babies), and quality of the connective tissues affect the stability of the pelvis. As pregnancy progresses up to 33 per cent of women develop varying degrees of pelvic girdle pain (PGP), pelvic instability or pubic symphysis dysfunction. All of these terms refer to pregnancy-related pain and instability of the pubic symphysis (front of pelvis) and sacroiliac joints (back of pelvis) which may or may not be associated with low back pain.

Stabbing, shooting, dull, or burning pain focuses around the sacro-iliac joints, one or both buttocks, back of legs and pubic bones. Walking, twisting, and stair climbing are painful. Sometimes a clicking or grinding is felt in the pubic bone, making walking difficult after standing. The discomfort is worse at night lying on the back, turning over in bed or lifting legs to get out of bed. Women with combined low back and PGP suffer more disability, often needing a walking stick or crutches to stay mobile.

Studies of pregnant women with PGP show they have dysfunction in their PF muscles, indicating specific PF muscle training is a crucial component in gaining relief of this condition.

To manage pelvic girdle pain:

- Avoid sitting with crossed legs, on the floor, or in the yoga lotus pose. When the pubic symphysis is painful, avoid straddle stretches or bike riding, which further opens the joint.
- Wear a support garment, or a sacro-iliac belt (above the pubic bone) to decrease sacro-iliac joint movement. Wear it to bed if pain disturbs your sleep.
- Side-sleep with a body pillow to support the abdomen and legs.
- Squeeze knees together to roll out of bed or get out of the car.
- Improve posture by growing tall and lengthening

through the top of the head. Regularly realign working and daily postures.

- Choose upright chairs with a cushion for lower back support; keep a cushion in the car to support the lower back curve.
- Lift the pelvic floor before coughing or sneezing, and stay upright instead of bending forwards.
- Avoid strenuous work and heavy lifting, eg: carrying bags of groceries or an older child.
- Avoid lying on the back for sex; try a side-lying position. Sex is too painful when PGP is severe.
- Wear low-heeled shoes (no higher than 3-4 cms) to reduce strain on the low back, pelvic and lower leg joints.
- Avoid exercises involving bouncing or balancing on one foot.
- Sit to pull on underwear, socks and trousers.
- Use massage and local heat to relax tight muscles.
- Sleep on a sheepskin for comfort with a pillow between the knees.
- Seek early treatment of PGP from a womens health physiotherapist to learn postural control and lumbopelvic stability exercises.

Low Back Pain

Low back pain differs from PGP with pain focused in the low back above the sacrum. It is similar to non pregnant low back pain with restricted low back movement, pain on forward bending and tenderness over spinal muscles and ligaments. Severe or persistent low back pain requires further investigation. Protect your spine and avoid lower backache during pregnancy with the following suggestions.

- Adopt a tall posture when sitting, standing and walking to regain and hold the gentle low back curve.
- Check sitting posture at the computer. Choose a chair that supports thighs with weight evenly distributed on sitting bones under the buttocks. Stand and move about frequently. Check chair height and optimal computer positioning on the desk. Details are available at www.ergonomics.com.au
- Engage in gentle exercise such as walking, swimming, tai chi, pregnancy yoga or aqua natal classes to ease spinal discomfort (modify the exercises if you have severe PGP).
- Exercises prescribed for non-pregnant women with back pain may need to be modified for pregnancy.
- Stop strenuous daily activities and heavier lifting, particuarly in a forward bent, twisting action to avoid excessive strain on lumbar spinal joints.
- Bend both knees to lift: keep a straight back (bottom out with chest lifted engages strong spinal muscles), and use the knack to lift PF muscles.
- Exercise pelvic floor, core and abdominal muscles regularly to reduce and control low back pain.
- Wear a support garment. The BellyBra is a full torso support undergarment designed to provide gentle support for the lower back and abdomen after 26 weeks. A wide elastic band sits below the tummy to

support the weight of the baby while the back stretch panels support the spine and improve posture. www.bellybra.com

- The newer SRC support garment provides support and compression to the pelvis, pelvic floor and thighs, whilst simultaneously supporting the hips and lower back. A reinforced gusset helps to compresses vulval varicosities. www.recoveryshorts.com.au

- Wear shoes with a lower heel to avoid the pelvis from tilting further forwards. Foot discomfort is related to baby and maternal weight gains. Additional pressure on supporting structures under the foot lowers the arches, adding to their length and width. Regular foot massages and orthotics arch supports bring relief.

- Use heat or ice packs and massage to alleviate spinal muscle tension. Side-lie for massage when the baby bump prevents lying face down. Some clinics provide a special pregnancy table to accommodate a pregnant tummy.

- To reduce low back pain; relaxation, massage, stretching, joint mobilization, improved body awareness and specific lumbo-pelvic stabilising exercises are effective.

Diastasis Rectus Abdominis

Diastasis rectus abdominis (DRA) is a midline split of the rectus abdominis muscles at the linea alba, which commonly occurs during mid to later pregnancy. The central linea alba anchors all the abdominal muscle layers and stretches and widens as baby grows. The gap usually occurs around the umbilicus but can spread upwards to the sternum or lower to the pubic bone.

Researchers report that as pregnancy progresses, 27 per cent of women develop a separation and by later pregnancy, 66 per cent are affected. It is more common in multi-parous, multi birth, caesarean and non-exercising mothers and associated with back pain and pelvic floor dysfunction.

Back pain and altered postures occur as the separation reduces the abdominals ability to stabilise the trunk. Prolapse, stress and faecal incontinence later in life are associated with a DRA, so protect the abdominals from excessive strain during pregnancy.

Avoid the following actions to reduce midline strain.

- Traditional abdominals-sit ups, crunches, double leg raises.
- Pilates exercises with neck/trunk flexion holds e.g. the '100's' exercise, plank holds, push ups.
- Fitball curl ups or backward stretches over the ball.
- Some yoga poses e.g. wheel and boat poses.
- Lifting or carrying heavy objects e.g. furniture, toddlers.

To protect the midline:

- Wear an abdominal support.
- Hand-support the abdomen during sneezing and coughing.
- Lift the pelvic floor to switch on core muscle support.

Review the test for DRA and postpartum treatment on page 106.

Pelvic Heaviness

If pelvic floor supports were stretched during previous pregnancies or damaged during an earlier birth, they will not be as effective in supporting the uterus during subsequent pregnancies. When the uterus sits lower in the pelvis, feelings of vaginal or pelvic discomfort and heaviness, genital swelling and urine loss may occur.

- Ask your doctor to determine if a pelvic organ has prolapsed or descended into the vaginal walls. Refer to prolpase on page 124.
- Fitting a vaginal pessary support reduces pelvic organ prolapse.
- Wear a support garment.
- Continue regular PF muscle strengthening.
- Avoid lifting or standing for long periods of time.
- Try swimming for exercise (water supports the heavy uterus).

Exercise during Pregnancy

The American College of Obstetricians and Gynecologists (ACOG) recommends women with low-risk pregnancies participate in moderately intense physical activity for 30 minutes or more daily, on most days of the week. If you are enjoying a problem-free pregnancy, and regularly exercised before pregnancy, continue to exercise with modified intensity.

An expanding abdomen changes the body's centre of gravity, so it's normal to feel less steady and slow down after 28 weeks. If you experience pain or conditions preventing physical activity, seek early advice, as it is important to keep moving throughout pregnancy.

Moderate exercise during pregnancy builds endurance in supporting muscles, making it easier to counteract the changing centre of gravity. Even light exercise pumps the heart faster, oxygenates body tissues and organs, stretches muscles, manages weight gain and helps with birth preparation. Suitable activities include walking, swimming, pre natal yoga, belly dancing, easy fitball exercises, Tai Chi, lightweights and gentle exercise classes. Consult caregivers for advice and guidelines if you are about to start a new exercise routine during pregnancy.

Marked changes occur in the cardiovascular and respiratory systems during pregnancy. Moderating activity or sport avoids overexertion and overheating and prevents sharp rises in heart and breathing rates.

The heart works 30 to 50 per cent harder during pregnancy, and the number of breaths taken per minute increases, especially after 28 weeks. Use the "talk test" to monitor exercise intensity. If you can still talk while exercising, you are working at an appropriate level. Not being able to talk due to fatigue or 'shortness of breath' indicates the intensity is too high. Adjust the exercise level lower or rest before recommencing at reduced intensity.

Use a heart rate monitor or manually check the heart rate during exercise (with finger tips over pulse points), to follow the research guidelines (over page) for recommended heart rates during exercise.

In fit pregnant women:

> Ages 20-29, 140 to 160 BPM (beats per minute)

> Ages 30-39, 140 to 156 BPM

> Ages 40+, 125 to 140 BPM

In lower fitness level pregnant women:

> Ages 20-29, 129 to 144 BPM

> Ages 30-39, 128 to 144 BPM

An ideal, balanced exercise program for pregnant women includes the following types of exercise.

Aerobic

Walking, swimming, belly dancing, or cycling for lung and heart fitness and weight control. Exercising in water supports the weight of the uterus, reduces the risk of joint and pelvic floor strain, prevents over heating and relieves swelling due to the effect of water's hydrostatic pressure against the skin. Changing from land to deep water running in a pool allows runners to continue impact free running and prevent pelvic floor and joint strain.

Strength and Balance

Prenatal yoga, modified Pilates, seated fit ball exercises; lighter weights and stretch band exercises improve and maintain muscle bulk and strength, while challenging balance control. These activities focus on slow controlled movement to strengthen PF and core muscles, both during pregnancy and after baby is born. Review the exercises from page 56.

If you did not exercise regularly before pregnancy, start with an easy activity such as walking, 4 or 5 days a week for 10 minutes, gradually increasing the time up to 30 minutes.

Running during pregnancy is too challenging for pelvic floor supports (due to hormonal changes in collagen and connective tissues) and runners are advised to walk or deep-water run to avoid strain.

Exercise Precautions

When exercising, remember to:

- Stretch slowly after exercise, but not excessively as pregnancy hormones increase ligament and tendon flexibility.
- Avoid bursts of high intensity or strenuous exercise and lower the intensity as pregnancy progresses.
- Avoid bouncing activities; wear a supportive sports bar during exercise.
- Wear a support garment to reduce PGP, and avoid exercise with body weight on just one leg.
- Avoid lying on your back to exercise beyond the 20th week.
- Eat healthy carbohydrates before exercising and sit down if you start to feel light headed.
- Stop exercising if tired or fatigued; pregnancy is not the time to overdo activity.
- Avoid overheating by exercising in the early morning, indoors, or in water (below 30 degrees Celsius); stay cool and drink plenty of water.
- Avoid lifting heavy weights, especially overhead

in later pregnancy. Strength training with light to moderate weights should be individually assessed.

- Avoid sit-ups, curl-ups or strenuous abdominal exercises to prevent more strain on the rectus abdominis midline and linea alba.
- Take a break from contact sports and sports with a higher risk of falling e.g. touch football, hockey, skiing and horse riding.

Avoid aerobic exercise if any of these conditions are present:

- dizziness, severe anaemia
- severe joint, pelvic or abdominal pain
- uncontrolled type 1 diabetes, thyroid disease, serious respiratory or cardiovascular disorders
- uncontrolled high blood pressure, pre-eclampsia (related to increased blood pressure and protein in the urine)
- incompetent cervix, placenta partially covering the cervix
- under developed foetus, multiple foetuses
- premature labour, cramping, pre-term rupture of membranes or leaking fluid, vaginal bleeding
- sudden swelling of ankles, feet or hands, morbid obesity

For exercise guidelines during pregnancy:
www.acog.org/publications/patient_education/bp119.cfm
www.noah-health.org/en/pregnancy/nine/fitness.html

Perineal Massage

Research shows women giving birth for the first time can reduce the risk of muscle tears and stitches by practicing regular perineal massage in the last four to six weeks of pregnancy (it does not always prevent tearing.) Massaging the perineum lets you experience some of the stretching and pressure sensations experienced during the crowning stage of birth when PF muscles are under maximal stretch during the passage of baby's head.

Perineal massage has two benefits: it increases the extensibility of PF muscles before labour, and you learn to relax PF muscles under stretch, in preparation for when baby's head applies strong opening pressure to the floor. Muscles and tendons are more at risk of tearing when the muscle suddenly contracts against a stronger force.

Keeping the pelvic floor open during the full stretch of the crowning head (while the uterus contracts with a powerful downwards pressure) is a significant part of reducing the risk of perineal tearing.

Practice the following perineal massage techniques or ask your partner for help, if you both feel comfortable. Seek midwife advice if unsure or you require further instruction.

- Wash hands and trim nails.
- Relax in a warm bath or apply hot towels to relax the PF muscles.
- Apply cold pressed oil or non petroleum based lubricant to the perineum (between the vagina and anus).

- Massage while squatting in front of a mirror or propped up in bed. Place both thumbs about 3 to 4 centimetres into the vaginal opening, just above the perineum.
- With thumbs hooked inside the vagina, slowly stretch down towards the anus and out to each side until you feel a stretching, tingling sensation. This opening action stretches the skin and muscle in the same way the baby's head stretches it during birth. Avoid the urethral opening during massage.
- Feel yourself 'letting go' as the perineum is stretched open rather than reacting by tightening and closing the PF muscles. Breathe with a relaxed jaw.
- Initially hold the stretch for 30 seconds then relax for a minute. Increase the stretch time up to 90 seconds over the next few weeks. Repeat several time, once or twice a day after 36 weeks of pregnancy.
- Do not perform perineal massage if herpes or other sexually transmitted disease is present.

Birth Classes

Many different organisations run classes and childbirth educators come from a variety of educational backgrounds such as doulas, midwives and physiotherapists.

Classes should cater for the various options women and their partners may choose or face, regardless of how they give birth. Educators are most effective when they offer classes flexible enough to suit your needs and don't impose their own personal beliefs on labour and birth.

Topics covered should include:

- Prenatal development, pregnancy diet, physical and emotional care.
- Precautions during pregnancy and premature labour.
- Different choices for birthing.
- What to expect during labour and birth.
- Breathing skills and positions to assist birth.
- Pain relieving techniques, pain relief options and interventions used.
- Developing a birth plan and knowing your rights when giving birth.
- Addressing fears about birth.
- Information on unexpected outcomes.
- Breastfeeding information.
- Caring for baby, baby massage and sleep techniques.
- Advice on early parenting skills including general baby care, baby massage and sleep techniques.

Birth and the Pelvic Floor

It is natural to be concerned about how birth may affect PF muscles, bladder, bowel control, and sexual function. Understanding what can harm the integrity of your pelvic floor, knowledge of birth procedures, positions, the choice of caregiver and the birth setting, all influence your pelvic floor outcome.

Pelvic floor damage with birth and ongoing problems are related to:

- poor birthing positions
- forced pushing with breath holding

- forceps or vacuum extraction
- third- and fourth-degree perineal tears
- a second stage longer than two hours
- mothers age (over 35) with first birth
- baby weighing over 4000 grams or malpositioned
- epidural anaesthesia
- episiotomy
- poor connective tissue

A breech presentation is where baby's bottom half presents first into the birth canal as opposed to the head. Breech vaginal birth is no longer recommended for first time mothers. During late pregnancy, external manipulation may be used to turn baby into the head down (vertex) position.

Some babies present posteriorally (with their back against their mother's back) instead of anteriorally, and while the majority turn to the front during labour others remain in the posterior position. This presentation usually slows birth particularly for first time mothers due to pressure of baby's head on the sacrum.

> *Before birthing, talk to your doctor or midwife about avoiding the routine use of interventions that increase the risk of pelvic floor disorders.*

Beforehand, ask your birth attendants about birthing positions and options to lessen pelvic floor damage. If labour is proceeding well, avoid lying on your back to birth. This position prevents the sacrum from slightly opening during second stage, making episiotomy more likely.

Choose side lying if you become exhausted or interventions are necessary. Talk to your midwife about different gravity assisted birthing positions, or a water birth.

Unnecessary cutting prior to birth of the baby's head can lead to more severe tearing. Cutting and stitching through the PF muscles leads to muscle wasting and weakness. A review of 177 research papers shows, 'The routine use of episiotomy to prevent severe perineal tears, urinary incontinence, faecal incontinence and genital prolapse should be abandoned'.

Researchers who looked at how women birthed and then related this to their subsequent pelvic floor problems, state, 'At least some of the less desirable outcomes attributed to vaginal births have been due to obstetric practices that are in need of improvement. Routine and overuse of episiotomy, routine use of epidurals, prolonged closed glottis pushing, lithotomy and other non-physiologic positions for birth all will cause differential increases for vaginal birth in the very perineal and pelvic floor problems to which this review has been directed. If these and other obstetric practices were improved, the reported differences between vaginal birth and caesarean section pelvic floor outcomes would likely narrow substantially'.

Women whose pelvic floor remains intact are less likely to suffer vaginal pain during intercourse. Birthing with episiotomy, significant tears and the use of forceps or suction, is associated with a higher frequency and severity of pain with intercourse at six months postpartum.

Women who birth vaginally have a higher rate of stress incontinence and vaginal prolapse than those who birth by elective caesarean. Research shows major muscle damage occurring with vaginal childbirth is associated with vaginal prolapse and is related to the use of forceps and suction. When unnecessary interventions are minimised, so are the adverse outcomes, which may encourage women to view vaginal births more positively.

For more information about preventing pelvic floor damage when giving birth:
www.childbirthconnection.org/article.asp?ck=10208.

Women who choose to birth by elective caesarean minimise the risk of major PF muscle damage and tearing. The likelihood of urge incontinence after the age of 50 is no different between women who had a caesarean or a vaginal birth. A caesarean birth is no guarantee of a problem-free pelvic floor. One study showed the prevalence of stress or urge incontinence and intravaginal prolapse was 42 percent in women with one or more vaginal births, as opposed to 35 percent in women who had a caesarean birth. Women who are in labour prior to the decision to perform a caesarean sustain more pelvic floor problems than women who elect to have a caesarean birth.

Caesarean risks and complications associated with anaesthesia include: blood clots, pulmonary embolism, a low-lying placenta (previa) or placenta growing into the uterus (accreta), premature birth and wound infection. The risk of placenta previa and accreta directly increases with the number of previous caesarean sections.

After a caesarean, some women report a loss of sensation

or pain around the abdominal incision, scar issues and internal adhesions (bands of collagen produced as part of the healing process following surgery, infection, inflammation or trauma). Complications occur when adhesions bind internal structures which are not normally connected. These fibrous links between pelvic or abdominal structures are likely to cause unusual pain and dysfunction. Reduced fertility related to post caesarean adhesions affects approximately 10 per cent of women.

Specific soft tissue mobilization helps to resolve scar or adhesion problems. This is best done by a professional therapist. **Always gain clearance from your surgeon before starting scar massage.**

Rebuilding strength in the pelvic floor and abdomen is just as important following a surgical birth as it is following a vaginal birth. To learn more about caesarean birth and vaginal birth after a previous caesarean, visit www.canaustralia.net

Case Study

Maria, 38 years, birthed her only child by caesarean four years earlier, and described increased frequency of lower back pain and bladder urgency. Maria had not exercised her PF muscles pre- or postpartum. She was unable to flatten her slack lower abdomen and had less feeling around the scar line. She stopped exercising because of embarrassment over her bulging abdomen and gained more weight. Bowel function had slowed and she strained with constipation. On examination, I found Maria was unable to lift her pelvic floor and activate the deep abdominal muscle corset, and her pelvic floor descended with coughing. Maria's low back was at risk of injury as the inner muscular corset failed to support her spine during daily activity.

After strengthening her pelvic floor and deep abdominal muscles, Maria reported no further bladder urgency. She achieved a flatter abdomen and relief of low back pain after four months of strength exercises and controlled eating. It became automatic for Maria to engage her PF muscles before lifting. Her bowel opened without straining (assisted by increased dietary fibre, water intake and a new toileting position) which lessened the downward stretching on her pelvic floor.

Stages of Birthing

These suggestions may help you during labour and birth to minimise pelvic floor injury.

During **Stage One** of active labour, the uterus is contracting to dilate the cervix to 7 centimetres. Take a shower or ask your partner to massage your back. Keep moving, rest, eat small meals and drink as needed.

During the **Transition Stage** the cervix opens to 10 centimetres to allow entry of the baby's head into the vagina. It can be the most intense stage of labour, lasting from a few minutes to several hours. Prepare your support team to provide lots of extra encouragement and attention during this time. Try changing positions onto all fours to reduce back discomfort. Visualise baby's head moving down and the cervix opening with each contraction. Breathe out with a relaxed jaw and low throat sounds.

Stage Two begins after full dilation of the cervix, when the uterus and vagina are continuous, allowing baby to leave the uterus and descend down to the pelvic floor. As the uterus contracts, it moves baby down the birth canal, so take it slowly and let the uterus do the work. As the contractions intensify, try different gravity-assisted positions until you find the most comfortable. If you become exhausted or interventions are required, lie on your side to birth.

Stage Three involves crowning and birth of baby. The perineum bulges with each push, as baby's head stretches pelvic floor muscles. When baby makes contact with the pelvic floor the involuntary urge to push is compelling and this effort, combined with uterine contractions, guides baby through the pelvic floor. During this time, you may be advised to slow the bearing down action to allow the perineum to stretch gradually without tearing.

The following suggestions may help to control and/or lessen muscle strain:

- Move to standing or kneeling on all fours so gravity assists baby's descent through the pelvis and down onto the pelvic floor. During this stage, your body may instinctively start to push.
- When pushing during a contraction, use the same opening action as when your bowel opens.
- Keep your jaw relaxed and breathe out with low throat sounds.
- If you feel dizzy or light headed, cup both hands over your mouth and rebreathe your carbon dioxide to relieve these sensations.
- A strong pressure sensation is felt as baby's head descends and presses on the rectum. It's not unusual to

lose small amounts of wind or bowel matter.

- When directed to stop pushing as baby's head crowns, use short 'har' throat sounds, then slowly birth baby's head to prevent tearing.
- Using a mirror lets you see the crown of baby's head and the progress made. Don't be discouraged if part of baby's head emerges then slips back. Birth of the head is close and it's normal for baby's head to move back slightly after each contraction.
- A helpful technique for the pelvic floor is to gently place your hand on baby's head and slowly 'breathe' baby out into your hand.
- Once baby's head is fully exposed, the head and body turns to one side to allow the shoulders and body to slip out.

Stage Four is placental delivery with uterine contractions and the urge to push resumes to separate the placenta from the uterine wall. This takes around 5 to 20 minutes following an injection of oxytocin. Without injection, natural placental delivery takes from 20 to 60 minutes.

Post Baby Pelvic Floor

Recovery following a vaginal or caesarean birth while settling into your role as a new mother can be challenging. This section contains information on postpartum issues and early recovery of pelvic floor and abdominal strength.

Bladder Control

Temporary loss of bladder control is common after vaginal

and caesarean birth. The most common type of postpartum weakness is from stress loss during sneezing, lifting and exercise, when exertion increases intra abdominal pressure. Research indicates that stress incontinence following first birth is a significant indicator of stress incontinence 12 years later.

Urge incontinence occurs when bladder muscles spasm, causing urine loss. You can control sudden bladder urgency by tightening the PC muscle, curling toes under and breathing until the urge passes. Ideally, the bladder should empty five or six times a day and once at night (depending on fluid intake), so persist with bladder training to delay emptying until you can hold at least 250mls before voiding. Months or years after birth, urgency can be related to untreated scar adhesions and muscular trigger points.

Urine flow is often heavier in the early postpartum days as the body eliminates excess pregnancy fluids. Occasionally, prolonged pressure from baby's head on the bladder during labour causes a temporary loss of bladder sensation in the first few days or weeks after the birth. If normal bladder signals are absent or urine does not release, inform medical staff immediately as a temporary urinary catheter is required to drain the bladder and prevent bladder distension.

Sitting on the toilet and relaxing the pelvic floor normally triggers bladder muscle contraction (these muscles are not under voluntary control). Toileting with abdominal tension prevents complete PF muscle relaxation and can lead to the habit of pushing down to pass urine (overriding the bladders normal action). Develop a healthy lifetime habit of voiding with abdominal wall relaxation in a tall sitting posture.

Weaker bladder control postpartum is effectively managed with regular PF exercises. Around 24-48 hours following an uncomplicated vaginal birth, start gentle PF muscle exercises to regain bladder control. If a catheter has been inserted to drain the bladder, begin gentle PF exercises after the catheter has been removed.

Even with good postpartum bladder control, add exercises to your daily heath plan so the pelvic floor copes with the demands of activity and lifting growing children, along with preventing incontinence and prolapse at menopause when hormonal changes lead to muscle thinning and weakening of urethral control. Women who practice regular PF exercises are more likely to retain strength of this muscle group into senior years.

When bladder or bowel weakness persists despite diligently repeating PF exercises, complete the bladder/bowel charts on page 149 and show the information to your medical team as incontinence rarely goes away by itself.

Skin, Perineal Muscle Tearing and Episiotomy

While it is common for first time mothers to sustain a minor, first-degree tear, the perineal area has a rich blood supply and heals quickly. Third and fourth degree tears are rare and more likely (but not always) to be associated with an extension of an episiotomy. Trauma (grazes and tears) to the anterior genitals affects the labia, front vaginal wall, urethra or clitoris. Injury to the posterior perineum affects the back vaginal wall, perineal muscles, anal sphincters and lining of the bowel. Bruising may occur to the genitals with a forceps or ventouse (vacuum) assisted birth.

There are different degrees of tearing:

- First degree tear involves injury to the skin.
- Second degree tear extends into the perineal muscles.
- Third degree tear extends into part of, or complete tearing of the anal sphincters.
- Fourth degree tear is a complete tear of the anal sphincters into the lining of the bowel.

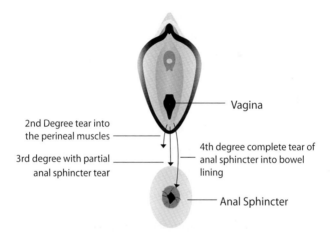

Fig. 15. Perineal Tears

Good hygiene prevents infection following a perineal tear or episiotomy. The following tips and treatment advice will help care for tears or stitches:

- If bladder sensation is poor or you cannot pass urine, try pouring water over the perineum. A catheter may be inserted to drain the bladder when other measures fail.
- Drink plenty of water and note if the bladder is

emptying easily and completely, and urine is pale.

- Use a urinary alkaliniser e.g. Ural, to reduce stinging when passing urine. Cranberry juice reduces the incidence of urinary tract infections.

- Be vigilant for signs of infection at the tear or stitch site. Pain, tenderness, redness, abdominal pain, difficulty urinating, thick discharge, offensive smell and fever are signs of infection, which require antibiotics.

Treatment

- Each time you urinate, fill a squirt (plastic sauce) bottle with warm water, squirt over the stitches and pat dry.

- Use ice packs over the stitched, swollen or bruised area or massage with an ice block immediately after the birth for 5 to 10 minutes every 2 to 3 hours for 48 hours or until swelling reduces.

- Spend 15 to 30 minutes lying down each day without the pad to promote healing. Sunbaths of 10 to 15 minutes are recommended for healing if you are assured of privacy!

- Start gentle PF muscle exercises to improve blood circulation, reduce swelling and speed up healing. Do 5 repetitions, 4 or 5 times daily. Moving around also improves circulation.

- Use a stool softener (2 teaspoons of Psyllium in water or juice twice daily), eat foods with higher fibre content (especially soluble fibre found in fruit, vegetables) and drink at least 6 glasses of water a day to keep stools soft.

- Some pain medication causes constipation. Rather

than risk further muscle damage from straining, ask your midwife for stool softeners while taking pain medication.

- Change pads frequently and do not use tampons, which can introduce bacteria.
- Hold a clean pad or folded toilet paper against your perineum to protect stitches during bowel opening.

Adding support to the perineum with bowel opening is important for all new mothers to reduce strain on recently stretched pelvic supports.

- Wear a firm pair of stretch briefs with a thick pad to keep pressure on the perineum.
- After the bowel empties, use wet wipes to clean the anal area from front to back.
- Avoid heavy lifting to minimise internal pressure increases down onto the pelvic floor.
- Use a soft cushion or pillow for comfortable sitting.
- Physiotherapists use ultrasound therapy over the perineum to reduce swelling.

Postpartum bleeding is typically constant for the first few days, then reduces to the regular menstrual loss. Light blood loss or spotting may continue for up to six weeks but this varies between women (may only be 2 to 3 weeks). Blood loss is augmented when breastfeeding helps to contract the uterus. Consult a midwife or doctor if you pass large clots or are concerned about blood loss. Use a mirror to check for redness, oozing or swelling around stitches and visit your doctor if signs of infection are present.

Anal Sphincter Tears

Poor wind and stool control, bowel urgency and painful intercourse are signs of anal sphincter damage that may not be detected postpartum. Around 11 per cent of women experience faecal incontinence at 3 to 6 months after vaginal or caesarean birth.

When the internal anal sphincter is affected, leaking of bowel content is uncontrolled (passive incontinence). A tear into the external anal sphincter leaves a woman unable to clamp the sphincter shut and prevent loss of faecal matter (stress and urge incontinence).

If you experience any loss of wind or stool control, urgency or chronic constipation, request an endoanal ultrasound (to detect internal and external sphincter tears) and consult a gastro-enterologist.

Treatment involves early repair of sphincter rupture (with a surgeon skilled in sphincter repair), antibiotics, PF exercises, biofeedback and stool softeners, or laxatives for easy bowel emptying. Sacral nerve stimulation is effective in the longer-term management of faecal incontinence. A small battery operated device inserted over the sacrum delivers impulses to the sacral nerves supplying the anal area.

Non-Surgical Early Treatment

- Reduce swelling by placing ice packs over the tear or repair for 10 to 15 minutes or use ice massage for 5 to 10 minutes, every 2 to 3 hours for 2 to 3 days.
- Take prescribed oral pain medication. Do not use pain medication in a suppository form inserted in the bowel.

- Lie down for breastfeeding and avoid lifting more than baby for 4-6 weeks.
- Take fibre or prescribed softeners and extra water to soften the stool as pain medication has a constipating effect on bowel contents.
- Use a handheld shower spray to clean around the anus after bowel empting.
- Avoid sitting on a rubber ring as the circle of pressure restricts blood flow to and from the stitched area and slows healing.
- Start pelvic floor exercises when comfortable.
- Make an appointment to see a midwife or women's health physiotherapist before leaving hospital for dietary advice, sphincter exercises and biofeedback in conjunction with surgical repair.

Anal Fissures and Haemorrhoids

The first two months postpartum are when anal fissures and haemorrhoids are likely to develop. These painful conditions are related to:

- Heavy birth weight babies.
- Traumatic labour or birth.
- Use of forceps during birth.
- Chronic constipation and difficulty fully emptying the bowel.
- Tearing of the tissues around the anus.

Treatment

- Soak in a warm bath several times a day (after stitches are removed). While in hospital small round tubs are placed in the toilet to take a mini bottom bath.

- Practice pelvic floor exercises and walk regularly.
- Avoid heavy lifting and prolonged coughing.
- Avoid straining or prolonged sitting to empty the bowel (use position on page 16).
- Use wet wipes (flushable wipes are now available) or a handheld shower spray to clean the anal area after the bowel empties. Toilet paper may be too abrasive to use.
- Treat constipation with a stool softener to reduce episodes of straining. Ask about a suitable non-chemical softener when breastfeeding or taking other medication.
- Ask your doctor or midwife about prescribing corticosteroid foam, cream or suppository to relieve pain, inflammation, swelling and itching.
- Combining medication with good anal hygiene and the listed suggestions will help shrink hemorrhoids and assist anal fissure healing.

Diastasis Rectus Abdominis

Diastasis Rectus Abdominis (DRA) is common after extreme abdominal wall stretching during pregnancy, and improves in the majority of mothers with a graduated return to controlled activity and exercise. In those affected, 53 per cent stay separated immediately postpartum and 36 per cent remain abnormally wide at 5 to 7 weeks postpartum.

Measure the diastasis by how many fingers fit into the separation. To check for separation:

- Lie on your back with both knees bent.

- Place fingers on the abomen at the umbilicus and lift your head off the floor.
- Look at how many fingers fit down into the gap.

A positive diagnosis of DRA is made when the separation stays wider than 1 finger width with abdominal contraction. A gap indicates more precautions and interventions are required. When the separation lasts longer than four weeks, it is associated with persistent lower back, pubic symphysis, sacroiliac joint pain, and incontinence. Wait 6 to 8 weeks after a caesarean before trying the head lift test (to allow for scar healing). A persistent gap will prevent the PF and transversus from generating sufficient compression force to stabilise the pelvis during activity.

The following suggestions will help to reduce the separation.

- With any degree of separation add compressive support to the abdominal muscles. Basic, low cost support is provided by a double layer of body-sized tubigrip or by wearing an abdominal binder. A smaller gap of 1 to 2 finger widths will benefit from compression for 4 to 6 weeks. When the gap is over 2 finger widths, compression may be needed for 4 to 6 months. The new SRC Recovery Shorts give full trunk support (up to the bra line) with pelvic floor support and abdominal compression. (see Resources, page 154).
- Roll onto your side to get in and out of bed to avoid sitting straight up and straining the separation.
- Add abdominal hand support when coughing or sneezing. Cross both arms over your abdomen with one hand on either side of the separated muscle. Pull the

hands and muscles towards the navel and hold with coughing or forward body movement.

- Lift the pelvic floor to switch on core muscles and decrease abdominal bulging before activity or exercise.
- See the physiotherapist before leaving hospital and seek postpartum treatment to manage and reduce the muscle separation.
- Avoid lifting and twisting actions e.g placing a toddler in a car seat. Move the feet to keep hips and shoulders facing in the same direction.
- Avoid heavy lifting and heavy housework for 12 to 16 weeks. Carry baby in front of the body, not to one side and stay tall when holding baby to avoid pelvic slumping.
- Stay committed to PF and core exercises to gain reduction of a DRA. The transversus abdominis is a corset like muscle that is crucial to abdominal rehabilitation. Lifting the pelvic floor contracts this muscle to flatten the abdominal wall, and stabilise the rectus separation.

Surgical repair may be necessary to improve function when the rectus muscles do not regain sufficient closure after 12 months and incontinence and/or low back pain persist. Diagnostic ultrasound is used to assess the extent of connective tissue damage before surgical correction with a surgeon experienced in this procedure.

Coccyx Damage

Occasionally, childbirth causes damage to the coccyx where

it attaches to the sacrum at the base of the spine. Some women report a 'popping' sound during birth and develop a painful coccyx postpartum. The coccyx doesn't actually break; it consists of two or three segments linked by ligaments and childbirth or a fall can strain the connections between these segments. Sitting forces the damaged joint apart causing pain. Seek treatment if coccyx pain is aggravated by PF exercises, or if the joint does not heal and remains painful.

Damage is more likely when body weight rests on the coccyx during birth, i.e. in a back lying or supported sitting position. These positions reduce the size of the pelvic outlet and increase the risk of damage or breaking open one of the little coccyx joints, by forcing it backwards when baby's head moves through the pelvis. Side lying, forward leaning positions and birthing in water (avoid sitting on the coccyx) allow all pelvic joints to gently stretch during labour.

Coccyx injury, pain and discomfort may last from 6 to 12 months. Some women report relief after focal injections, while others resort to having the coccyx surgically removed (this does not always resolve the problem and post operative complications are common).

Treatment

- Visit a doctor who specialises in coccyx injuries and a women's health physiotherapist to check the coccyx and sacral alignment. Muscle spasms and trigger points in PF muscles or buttock muscles attaching to the sacrum may be aggravating the coccyx pain and require myofascial release, stretching, dry needling or pain relieving injections.

- An x-ray or MRI scan will be suggested initially. Be sure to ask the radiographer for a clear view of the coccyx so it is included in the x-ray. Ask about a sit/stand dynamic x-ray to show if the coccyx is dislocating with sitting.
- Initially, use ice packs to reduce swelling along with anti-inflammatory and pain medication to relieve acute pain.
- Sit on a coccyx cushion to relieve pressure.
- Keep body weight over the sitting bones and the front pubic bone. It is usually more comfortable to sit in a slightly forward leaning position.
- Continually leaning the weight to one side may provoke back pain or bursitis around the hip taking the weight.
- Avoid sitting on the floor or on a hard plastic or wooden chair.
- In the car, use the coccyx cushion underneath and a small support cushion in the lower back.
- Avoid sitting for long periods; stand and move frequently.
- Keep bowel movements soft to avoid straining.
- Pain may be prolonged if the muscles controlling the bladder are weak or not working effectively postpartum. After inflammation reduces, learning to tighten and lift the PC muscle may ease pain for some sufferers in the short and long term. This action should be started gently to prevent aggravation of pain.
- Some women gain relief after a focal ganglion impar

block or injection into the sacrococcygeal junction by a doctor experienced in treating coccyx injuries.

Prolapse

Pelvic organs herniate or slip down into the vaginal walls when supporting pelvic ligaments weaken and PF muscles fail to close and lift. Prolapse occurs in 50 per cent of childbearing women and those with few symptoms may be unaware of this condition until a bulge presents at the vaginal entrance. Prolapse can affect one or more pelvic organs: the symptoms indicating specific prolapses are discussed on page 124.

Case Study

Leah, at 28, felt so healthy and happy after the birth of her second child, she was chopping and carrying timber for the winter fireplace three weeks afterwards. She was shattered when her cervix prolapsed down to the vaginal entrance.

Leah was restricted to lifting only her newborn son, and was fitted with a pessary support to reduce the prolapse while practising daily PF strength exercises. After five months of PF strengthening along with a Fitball program (no crunches) and stretch band exercises, Leah regained the strength of her internal muscular corset, allowing for pessary removal. Six months later, she reported no signs of prolapse but continued to be cautious about the amount of weight she lifted and committed to a lifetime of PF exercises.

Post Baby Blues

Post baby blues affect up to 80 per cent of new mothers in the first week after giving birth and usually disappear in a week or two. Getting more sleep and seeking help from family and friends is an effective way to overcome the blues. Symptoms of postnatal depression include feelings of anxiety, loss of interest in food, sex and other pleasurable activities, lasting longer than two weeks and occurring in the first year after giving birth. Typical feelings are exhaustion, tearfulness, loss of confidence, inability to cope, memory problems, and sleep and appetite changes. These feelings are related to hormonal imbalance, sleep deprivation, exhaustion, body changes and pelvic floor dysfunction.

Seek help and advice early from your health care provider, as there are many proven ways to overcome depression. Sleep, exercise, counselling, problem solving therapy, interpersonal psychotherapy, cognitive behavior therapy, massage, meditation, diet, fish oils and some supplements are effective proven treatments. Women with moderate to severe PMS (pre menstrual syndrome), a history of depression or have suffered previous postpartum depression are most at risk and require professional intervention.

When birth is traumatic or an unexpected caesarean section is performed, a 'post traumatic' reaction may occur. Women who experience an unexpected or unwanted caesarean may grieve for the loss of a vaginal birth leaving some feeling sad, anxious, violated and betrayed. The symptoms of any birth-related trauma can emerge weeks, months or even years after the event. Talk to your midwife about how you are feeling before going home.

If you or your partner become aware of any feelings associated with depression, seek help early from caregivers, to understand and overcome these feelings. Counselling and support groups help to resolve frustration, anger, grief or resentment. Involve your partner so they can offer physical and emotional support and begin to understand what you are going through. When new mothers develop depression, their partners also have a higher risk of developing depressive symptoms. For more information: www.panda.org.au or www.beyondblue.org.au

Case Study

Confident, sporty Kate, a 33 year-old psychologist, went from having confidence in her strong and active body to finding she no longer liked or trusted it since the birth of her son, Harry. Her faith was shaken when she could not join social activities with friends and joked, 'Harry has strained my wa-wa, and now I pee my pants'. Kate kept Ziploc bags with pads and fresh panties in her car, nappy bag and desk at work to cope with regular accidents. Harry was not the only one who needed changing through the day.

Forceps assisted Harry's birth after a prolonged second stage of labour. Kate had previously enjoyed a close, intimate sex life with her husband but now depression crept in as her relationship was affected by sexual dysfunction. Kate said, 'It felt like a switch had flicked off, making everything numb'.

From her psychologist's perspective, Kate wryly noted if any woman experienced prolonged sleep deprivation, loss of sexual sensation, wet pants and restricted activity (with resultant weight gain), depression was a certain outcome.

The turning point for Kate came when she discovered she was not exercising the right muscles. Once she found, coordinated and strengthened PF and core muscles, she quickly regained bladder control and orgasmic sensation returned. Her mood became more confident along with a new understanding of her body, and the effect of exercise on her pelvic floor.

Guidelines for Return to Exercise

Focus on walking and holding upright posture in the first weeks after birth, as you get in shape from 'the inside out' with pelvic floor and core exercises. Training these muscles first—to recover strength and coordination—is the number one priority before starting an aerobic, fitness or gym programme.

The following return to activity guidelines contain suggested timeframes for resuming aerobic activity. Resuming exercise depends on the new mother's level of fitness, exercise history, any injuries or complications with birth, and whether PF and core rehabilitation has been consistent and effective. Be wary of returning to 'bootcamp' style programmes and challenging exercise classes. Bootcamp is based on the Royal Canadian Air Forces 5BX and 10BX systems adopted for training military personnel, and is not suitable for new mothers.

- Birth to 16 weeks - Tall sitting, standing and walking, PF exercises, 'Train It' exercises and easy swimming after blood loss has ceased.
- 16 to 24 weeks - After an uncomplicated vaginal birth, return to postnatal exercise class and low impact aerobic activities e.g. swimming, water aerobics, tai chi or basic belly dancing and 'Train It' exercises.

- 24 weeks onwards - After an uncomplicated vaginal birth, modified yoga, basic pilates and fit ball classes with experienced postpartum instructors.

Following a caesarean or complicated vaginal birth, commence the 'Train It' program when you are comfortable. Gradually add easy activities as pain settles and your pelvis and trunk strengthen.

Delay returning to more challenging physical activity for up to 6 to 12 months if you experience any of the following: caesarean birth, third and fourth degree perineal tears, infection and further surgery, prolonged second stage labour with interventions, rectus diastasis separation, unresolved pelvic instability, coccyx damage, prolapse, or incontinence. Consult a women's health professional to safely guide return to activity according to your level of PF and core stability, strength and general fitness.

Running

Avoid high-impact activities in the first 16-20 weeks until joints are more stable and PF and core muscles are stronger. Running is not suitable as an early activity due to the stress on joints and the pelvic floor, and the potential to cause discomfort in lactating breasts (breastfeed prior to exercising).

Experienced runners benefit by focusing on PF and core exercises, before attempting running. Leaking towards the end of a long uphill walk or run indicates PF muscles are fatigued and require more training in their endurance and strength modes. Change from high-impact to low-impact exercise such as walking, swimming and easy dancing while continuing to strengthen pelvic control.

When runners resume their fitness program, I suggest they start by running for one to two minutes then walking for 10 to 15 minutes, and repeating this pattern while slowly increasing the running period and decreasing the walking period. Progress is guided by pelvic floor control rather than focusing on the running time. Only increase the run distance when the PF floor is coping at the current level. Don't rush back to running early postpartum as pregnancy weight gains add to stress on the pelvic floor and pelvic, hip and leg joints.

Stretch to maintain muscle length, however avoid strong, end range stretching to increase flexibility until 16 to 20 weeks postpartum when the effects of pregnancy hormones are minimal.

Postpartum Tips

- Walk for 30 to 60 minutes most days to burn calories and reduce weight. Adopt the tall posture when pushing the baby buggy or carrying baby in a sling or back pack.
- Eat generous servings of fruit, vegetables and lean protein to replace the empty calories in snack food.
- Visit a dietician or nutrutionist for eating guidelines if your breastfeeding appetite goes into overdrive.
- Complete PF strength exercises 3 times a day.
- Train inner muscles first, to recover strength and coordination for dynamic core and trunk stability.
- Avoid challenging abdominal exercises in the first six months postpartum to prevent strain on the rectus connective tissue.

- Wear a support garment for 4-6 weeks to control posture, support pelvic joints, compress pelvic organs and protect the rectus midline.
- Running is not advised before 16 to 20 weeks due to the added stress on joints and the pelvic floor.
- Deep water running burns calories and improves fitness without the impact loading on the pelvic floor and lower limb joints.

Recovery After Caesarean Birth

Healing after surgery (along with enjoying and caring for your newborn) is now a priority. Accept offers of help from friends and family. Let them know beforehand how much you would value the gift of a few hours of their time with cooking, baby sitting or housework. Recovery rates following a caesarean vary between women, taking up to six months for the deep abdominal muscle layers to fully heal. Allow time to regain abdominal strength and shape, and gently strengthen from the inside out with the Control It and Train It exercises (see page 43).

Following surgery, time is spent in recovery while vital signs stabilise. It takes hours for the anesthetic to wear off and for feeling to return to the lower body. Ask for a heated blanket if shaking starts in the recovery period. Sometimes an annoying pain is felt under the shoulder blade from air entering the abdominal cavity during surgery. Passing wind after surgery is a good sign showing the intestinal muscles are contracting to move wind out of the body. Wind pain is often experienced during the first few days (common after all abdominal surgery).

Occasionally headaches present after an epidural.

The first 24 hours are challenging due to the restrictions of a urinary catheter (to drain the bladder) and an intravenous drip to administer fluid, pain medication and antibiotics if needed. The catheter and drip are usually removed the next day, which makes moving around somewhat easier. Bladder incisions (not common during caesareans) require an indwelling catheter for 7 to 10 days and are associated with an increased risk of urinary tract infections. Report any pain or difficulty passing urine.

Some women report low levels of pain while others need regular pain relief and more support following a surgical birth. Complications, support received and emotional coping skills influence the level of pain experienced post-surgery.

To encourage urine flow, try a warm shower or pour water over the perineum to relax PF muscles. Drugs given during or after surgery for pain control can affect bladder and bowel function. Once the catheter is removed, empty the bladder every few hours for a day or two, as a full bladder may cause pressure and pain on the caesarean scar. Speak to the midwife or doctor if the regular sensations associated with a full bladder are not present.

The first bowel movement can be a bit scary, with natural concern about stress on the caesarean scar. Support the wound by applying gentle pressure with your hand while relaxing the abdomen and anal sphincter. Sitting tensed up on the toilet keeps the anal sphincter closed. As some pain relieving medication slows the bowel action, keep up water intake, eat fibre-rich foods and ask your midwife about stool softeners.

Vaginal blood loss is similar for both vaginal and caesarean births, and is checked for the amount and colour of the blood. Any significant blood clots should be reported. When baby is breastfed, their sucking stimulates the release of hormones, causing uterine contractions and increased blood loss. The flow also becomes heavier in standing, as gravity drains fluids from the uterus. It's normal to pass some blood clots but check with your midwife after any clots are passed. Light blood loss may continue for two to six weeks after the birth (this varies between mothers).

Caring for the Caesarean Scar

The sutured layers of uterus, connective tissues, and skin take time to heal. It is wise to delay returning to activity and restrict the everyday workload, to ensure healing is uninterrupted. Sutures hold the wound layers together while collagen repairs around the incisions. Abdominal muscles need time to repair before gentle strengthening can begin. During this time avoid any heavy activity to ensure the scar does not break down. The stitches dissolve later (or are removed) as tissue healing progresses.

Regularly check the scar for signs of infection: redness, pain, local areas of tenderness, offensive smell, swelling or oozing of fluid. Report this to your doctor immediately. Even though antibiotics are routinely given in theatre, infection can still develop after surgery.

Some women report numbness or hypersensitivity around the scar, which may take 12 to 24 months to regain normal sensation. Other women report patches of permanent numbness for years afterwards. As nerve re-growth is slow, sensation can take years to return post surgically.

The scar is purple after surgery and takes months to go from purple to pink to white, and pubic hair re-growth may partly cover the scar. Gentle massage promotes healing and helps to prevent adhesions from forming between the uterus and other organs, but only once the scar is suffciently healed. If massage is too firm or started too early, it will cause bleeding and slow down healing. *Do not commence scar massage until you have clearance from your surgeon.* Avoid Brazilian waxing until perineal or abdominal scars are fully healed and pain free.

Recovery Tips

- Within 24 hours you will be encouraged to get out of bed with assistance, if there are no complications. Usually, pain medication is routinely prescribed, but always ask if more pain relief is needed so these early adventures are more tolerable. A shower relaxes and freshens and walking upright helps to pass abdominal wind, improves circulation and reduces the risk of deep vein thrombosis.

- While resting in bed, start simple leg exercises to improve circulation. Pump both feet up and down and circle ankles regularly for 1 to 2 minutes.

- Take 5 deep lower rib expanding breaths every hour to restore full diaphragmatic movement (this was restricted during pregnancy).

- Bend both feet up towards your buttocks. Gently flatten the lower back into the bed then gently arch the lower back 5 to 10 times.

- Support the incision line with your palm while getting

out of bed and walking to the bathroom. Keep knees together, roll onto your side, and use the other arm to push up. Hold your abdomen when coughing or sneezing.

- Instead of strong coughing use 'repeated 'huffing' to dislodge any chest secretions to reduce the impact of strong coughing on the scar.

- It is safe to shower with a waterproof dressing and once the dressing is removed, gently run water over the incision line, but avoid using soap. Pat dry with a fresh towel. Sometimes silicone tape is placed over the incision and changed daily for 2 to 4 weeks to decrease scarring.

- Wear high-waisted knickers (Bridget Jones-style) to avoid the elastic waist rubbing on, or irritating the incision line.

- Place a pad over the incision line (stick to the knickers) to prevent them rubbing on the stitches.

- Standing in a slightly forward-bent posture takes tension off the scar but does not engage the PF and core postural muscles.

- Pay attention to 'tall' sitting, standing and walking postures to switch on core muscles. Breathe out as you sit or stand up into a 'tall' posture to engage the PF and core.

- Start gentle PF exercises to engage the deep abdominal muscle.

- Lift PF muscles before picking up baby.

Menopause and the Pelvic Floor

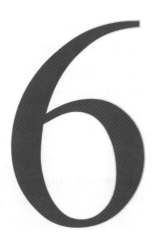

Menopause is officially confirmed when periods have stopped for 12 months. Some women first become aware of PF issues as lower oestrogen levels combined with less activity and weight gain prove to be the tipping point for pelvic floor control. This section contains some of the commonly reported changes affecting the pelvic floor.

Leaking When You Walk or Exercise

Urine loss with menopause is related to the drop in oestrogen levels causing softening of the urethral lining, in turn reducing the closing pressure of the urethral sphincters. Strengthening PF muscles will help improve closing pressure and prevent urine loss.

With weight gain, internal abdominal fat loads more pressure down onto the pelvic floor and contributes to poor bladder control and pelvic organ prolapse. Urine loss, perceived lack of time or poor self-esteem prevents some women from exercising. Commit to some form of exercise EVERY DAY to gain improvements in energy and mood, muscle and bone strength, glucose metabolism, sleep patterns and blood pressure.

> *Do not stop exercising if you leak. Continence guards inserted vaginally under the bladder neck can relieve urine loss while you exercise and strengthen PF muscles.*

If it seems difficult to get started, seek advice from a physiotherapist, exercise physiologist or trainer. Ask a friend to come along as a training 'buddy' to help you stay on track with regular exercise. Many clients tell me the unexpected benefit of having a dog is the discipline of daily walking.

Controlling weight gain at menopause is immmortant to avoid the fastest growing disease in the world – diabetes. Women who are both overweight and have Type II diabetes have a 50 to 70 percent increased risk of incontinence. Postmenopausal diabetic women are more likely to develop severe urinary incontinence and urinary tract infections. A recent study of pre-diabetic, overweight women showed the group who exercised and changed their diet reduced stress incontinence and the risk of developing Type II diabetes. To learn more about diabetes: www.diabetes.com.au

Prolapse

Lower oestrogen levels, weaker PF muscles and weight gains contribute to pelvic organ prolapse at menopause. The symptoms listed below are associated with the different types of prolapse which affect one or more pelvic organs.

A vaginal anterior or front wall prolapse (Fig. 16) occurs when the bladder and/or urethra descends into the front vaginal wall. Commonly reported symptoms are:

- urine loss with coughing and activity
- bulging at the front of the vaginal entrance with coughing
- tampons fall out
- bladder emptying problems
- incomplete emptying/recurrent bladder infections
- discomfort/pain during intercourse

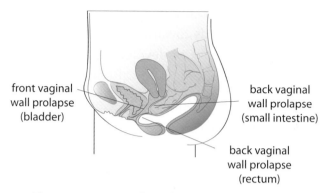

front vaginal
wall prolapse
(bladder)

back vaginal
wall prolapse
(small intestine)

back vaginal
wall prolapse
(rectum)

Fig. 16. Front and Back Vaginal Wall Prolapse

A vaginal posterior or back wall prolapse (Fig. 16) occurs when the rectum descends into the back vaginal wall with the following symptoms:

- difficult and/or incomplete bowel emptying requiring manual assistance
- straining to empty the bowel
- bulging at the back of the vaginal entrance with straining
- difficult to retain a tampon
- discomfort/pain with intercourse

When the small intestine descends into the upper back vaginal wall between the uterus and rectum, common symptoms are:

- constipation and difficult bowel emptying
- rectal pressure sensation
- lower back pain, worse after prolonged standing
- vaginal discharge or bleeding
- discomfort/pain with intercourse

Utero-vaginal descent occurs when the cervix (and uterus)

descends vaginally (Fig. 17). Women with a retroverted uterus (the uterus tips backwards towards the spine in 20 per cent of women) are more at risk of developing an advanced stage of this prolapse and requiring surgical correction. Symptoms include:

- urinary incontinence
- constipation
- low back pain
- vaginal/pelvic heaviness
- menstrual type cramps
- painful intercourse

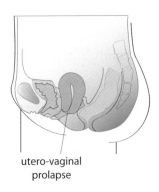

utero-vaginal
prolapse

Fig. 17. Utero-vaginal prolapse

Vaginal vault prolapse affects women who have previously had a hysterectomy. The upper part of the vagina sags down into the vagina and may descend externally. Common symptoms include:

- vaginal pressure
- painful intercourse
- back pain
- urinary incontinence

Rectal prolapse occurs when the rectum prolapses through the anus, due to nerve damage with chronic straining, diarrhea or multiple sclerosis, and is more common with advancing age. Another form of prolapsed rectum is called internal intussusception, where the upper rectum slides down inside the rectum like a tube within a tube.

Risk of prolapse

White and Latina women have the highest rate of prolapse followed by Asian and African-American women. If your mother had a prolapse, your risk increases three-fold. There is an increased risk around menopause for women with several children and a larger waist measurement. Chronic bowel straining, coughing with chest disease, heavy lifting and over-challenging exercise set the scene for prolapse. If the second stage of labour was prolonged, forceps or suction was required or the first time mother was over 35, the risk of prolapse is increased. Large uterine fibroids, pelvic tumors and excessive abdominal weight place more internal pressure down onto pelvic organs, requiring more supportive effort from the PF muscles.

Non-surgical treatment

An internal exam is performed to determine the type of prolapse and you will be asked to bear down to see how this pressure affects the prolapse. An ultrasound or magnetic resonance imaging (MRI) test may be ordered to determine the degree of prolapse.

Prolapse does not go away by itself and not all cases of prolapse require surgery. Many women respond to lifestyle changes, PF muscle strengthening and vaginal oestrogen combined with a pessary support. This is a ring shaped device inserted vaginally to reduce and relieve prolapse symptoms and prevent the prolapse from worsening. Many different types are available and your doctor will select and fit the most appropriate pessary for the type of prolapse. Fitting is by trial and error and it is not unusual to change the size or type a few days or months later. Fitting is generally unsuccessful for women who present with absent sacral reflexes, a higher stage of prolapse, a genital hiatus greater than 4cm or who cannot lift their pelvic floor.

Some surgeons insert a pessary to relieve symptoms while waiting for surgery or if surgery is not possible due to existing medical conditions. Instructions for pessary management include returning to your doctor every 3 months for removal, cleaning, vaginal wall inspection and refitting. Some women prefer to remove their pessary at night and reinsert in the morning. Pessaries are used in younger women to relieve incontinence, support an incompetent pregnant cervix or reduce prolapse after childbirth. Oestrogen cream is used in conjunction with the pessary to improve the quality of the vaginal tissues and improve muscle tone in menopausal women.

Not all prolapses improve with only PF exercises. If there is significant connective tissue, muscle or nerve damage, surgery is the treatment of choice. Your surgeon may do brilliant work, but continuing to lift heavy weights, straining to empty the bowel and failing to control posture or strengthen a weak pelvic floor, puts you at risk of further prolapse after surgery. Following initial surgical repair of a prolapse, there is a 30 percent chance of failure. Studies show after one year, successful pessary treatment is as effective as surgery. A long-term follow-up study is underway to determine if the results are lasting.

There are ways to reduce your risk of prolapse (and re-prolapse):

- Sit, stand and walk tall by lengthening up through the crown of your head to keep pelvic floor and core muscles active.
- Use the 'knack' to lift PF muscles before coughing or sneezing.
- Avoid lifting more than 4-5 kg or shifting furniture.
- Reduce bowel strain (a common cause of prolapse). Eat fibre rich food and drink up to two liters of water daily to keep stools soft. Use a fibre rich emulsion such as fibogel or metamucil to soften stools.
- Treat a chest infection or allergic sneezing early to avoid prolonged coughing or sneezing.
- Commit to a regular PF muscle strengthening program. Avoid pushing yourself in group exercise classes, as PF muscles may fail under the load of challenging exercises.
- Reduce your waist circumference to lighten the internal pelvic floor loading.
- Consider learning slow belly dancing or slow latin dance to develop control and strength in pelvic and abdominal muscles. Progress to faster movements after muscle control improves.

Bladder Urgency

An urgent bladder repeatedly sends signals to empty, increasing toilet visits to avoid accidents. This can change the way you plan your day, noting the location of every toilet before going shopping and avoiding long trips on public transport. Turning on the tap, putting a key in the door or heading to the toilet increases urgency and leaking. Getting out of bed in the morning and leaking on the way to the bathroom is hardly the best way to start your day!

Urgency may indicate the PC muscle is not effectively closing the sphincters around the urethra and the base of the bladder. This muscle is your body's inbuilt system to control urgency. Learning to lift and strengthen the PC at the front of your pelvic floor will help to control urgency and urine loss.

Ask your doctor for a midstream urine test to exclude infection as a cause of urgency and leaking. Other causes of urgency include urethral diverticulum, interstitial cystitis, hyperactive PF muscles, trigger points, pelvic adhesions and pain syndromes.

> *Bladder urgency after exercise or heavy work is a warning sign the PF muscles are not supporting the bladder and pelvic organs.*

Urgency after exercise or heavy gardening, indicates the level of exercise is too difficult, the PF muscles are tiring and unable to control internal pressure. A strong, coordinated pelvic floor lifts to counter the rise of internal pressure during activity and exercise. Keep strengthening PF muscles, ask about easier exercise options and avoid heavier garden tasks.

Quieten bladder urgency by curling your toes under, lifting the pelvic floor, relaxing your waist and breathing for ten seconds or until urgency passes. Walk to the toilet when urgency is controlled.

Urinary Tract Infections

Lower oestrogen levels leave women more prone to urinary tract infections (UTI) around menopause. When the bladder does not completely empty, residual urine is an easy home for infection.

To help prevent intercourse related UTI, use vaginal oestrogen cream and a vaginal lubricant to reduce discomfort during intercourse. Find a natural product without chemicals, preservatives (parabens) or stabilisers, which disrupt the vagina's natural flora. Glycerine may increase the risk of vaginitis and parabens may have an oestrogenic effect. Go natural and use olive, sesame, or sunflower oils externally (if using condoms, opt for the oil resistant non-latex variety).

Habits to prevent frequent UTI's

- Drink more water to flush out the urinary system and remove bacteria.
- Use urinary alkalisers to relieve burning symptoms.
- Avoid caffeine and artificial sweeteners, as some cause urgency. Diet soft drinks contain a double bladder whammy of caffeine and artificial sweeteners.
- Take cranberry tablets or juice to prevent E. coli bacteria from attaching to urethral and bladder walls and triggering a UTI. These bacteria cause 85 percent

of infections. Women with interstitial cystitis report cranberry aggravates UTI pain.

- Avoid douches and vaginal sprays to prevent urethral irritation. If urine loss causes a rash, use a simple baby barrier cream or pawpaw ointment. Use pads designed for urine loss rather than menstrual fluids. Avoid using talcum powder near your pelvic floor.

- Before and after intercourse, wash the pelvic area to reduce bacteria. Insist on an equal level of hygiene from your partner.

- After intercourse, empty your bladder. Avoid intercourse positions which direct thrusting towards the front vaginal wall where the urethra is situated.

- After bowel emptying, always wipe from front to back. Wash the anal area or carry a pack of wipes to prevent the E. coli bacteria from migrating forward to the urethral entrance. Tampon strings can pick up the E. coli bacteria and transfer them forwards to the vagina and urethra.

- Strengthen PF muscles. Improving muscular support helps the bladder to fully empty.

- Your doctor can arrange a simple post-void ultrasound to determine whether the bladder is emptying fully.

Most women who develop a UTI require antibiotic medication to quickly settle the symptoms.

If frequency, burning and pain above your pubic bone is present, even when your midstream urine tests free of bacteria, the cause may be interstitial cystitis (IC), painful bladder, urethral diverticulum or triggered by other painful mechanisms associated with IC. Tight PF muscles and painful trigger points causing UTI-type pain are common in these women, who gain relief with treatment of the tight muscles and painful trigger points. For more information: www.ichelp.org

Urethral Diverticulum

Lack of knowledge about urethral diverticulum has led to this relatively common condition remaining undiagnosed in women with chronic genitourinary conditions. Previously, women with recurrent infections, retro pubic pressure, post-void dribbling and painful sex (without vaginal infection or cystitis), were given the blanket diagnosis of 'urethral syndrome'.

The urethra is surrounded by microscopic paraurethral glands concentrated around the lower third of the urethra, that drain into the Skene Ducts, adjacent to the urethral opening. Infection in these glands is relatively common and under diagnosed. This condition is diagnosed by various imaging techniques and careful pinpoint palpation of the urethra, through the front vaginal wall.

If you have a history of the symptoms associated with paraurethral gland infection, use your index finger to carefully palpate the sides of the urethra 2 to 3 centimeters up along the front vaginal wall. Specific tenderness is an indicator of paraurethral gland infection. Sometimes 'milking' the urethra releases the build up of infected fluid. Relapses may occur months or years later and are again confirmed with urethral palpation through the vaginal wall.

Treatments for urethral diverticulum symptoms include

surgical excision of periurethral tissue, internal urethral cutting procedures and forceful urethral dilation. These procedures may be associated with ongoing pain, incontinence and recurring symptoms. Antibiotics are effective for acute infection and muscle relaxants may be prescribed to reduce muscle spasms.

Muscular overactivity is a natural reaction of pelvic floor muscles to pain, infection and urine loss. Hot baths bring soothing relief of muscle spasm. Treatment with a women's health physiotherapist is indicated when pelvic floor muscles are chronically tight.

Changes to your Sex Drive

Some menopausal women are dismayed to discover they have less desire for sex and do not respond to the same triggers or turn-ons which worked in the past. Sex is as much an emotional as a physical sensation for women; it is complex and involves the mind-body connection. The common physical symptoms affecting a woman's sexuality are:

- Vaginal dryness – decreased vaginal blood supply and thinner vaginal walls cause discomfort with intercourse. This can be relieved by using oestrogen cream or a vaginal lubricant and moisturiser. (e.g. Replens).
- Bladder control – weaker urethral closing pressure may result in loss of urine during sex. This weakness improves with pelvic floor muscle strengthening, combined with vaginal oestrogen cream or pessary tablets.

- Night or day sweats – these hot episodes put a dampener on romantic feelings and may require the fan or air conditioner on full blast.

- Low libido – some women experience great frustration and a sense of loss or grieving because their bodies are changing (without their permission). It is a life stage when women are often juggling working and parenting roles, financial and relationship issues and perhaps caring for ageing parents. It is important both partners understand the physical and emotional changes of menopause. Express any concerns to your partner and enjoy discovering different ways to make your sex life more pleasurable and fun. Even when libido levels change, women don't lose their need for affection, emotional closeness and intimacy.

It may be too simplistic to 'medicalise menopause' and try to find a 'cure' for loss of sexual desire with hormone replacement therapy (HRT). Women who lose their sexual desire as they age might be reacting to their own body image rather than to hormonal changes. The less attractive a woman thinks she is, the more likely she is to report a decline in sexual desire. Some women discover their sex drive improves when the declining levels of oestrogen, progesterone, androgens (including testosterone) are restored. There is ongoing disagreement and confusion over the use of HRT, however some women genuinely gain an improved quality of life, with marked relief of hot flushes, mood swings and vaginal dryness. Some studies on HRT show it can worsen urinary incontinence in some women and cause incontinence in previously unaffected women.

In *The Secret Pleasures of Menopause,* Dr Christiane Northrup reminds women their brain is the biggest and most important sex organ in their body. She encourages women to pursue activities they love, bring them pleasure and connect them with their inner joy: '...before you can have a passionate relationship with someone else, you have to already be in a passionate relationship with yourself and your life.'

Dr. Christiane Northrup's book *The Wisdom of Menopause* contains a wealth of knowledge to guide women through this transitional life stage. I recommend both books. Visit her website at www.drnorthrup.com

Changes in vaginal sensation, arousal and orgasm intensity may occur postpartum, after pelvic surgery or with menopause. Many women with altered sexual response suffer silently, unaware of treatment options including the link to poor PF muscle control. They feel deeply embarrassed over loss of urine or wind, or if their partner comments on less sensation during intercourse. A weak pelvic floor allows air into the vagina during intercourse with embarrassing wind noises. Major illness, depression and some medications also lessen desire and vaginal lubrication.

Understanding female sexual anatomy will help you realise how sexual response and orgasm intensity relate to PF muscle strength, and why surgery has the potential to affect sexual response.

Female Sexual Anatomy

Most anatomy books display the external female genitalia (with the clitoris shown externally as a pea sized bump) along with the internal organs, and omit internal sexual anatomy. The clitoral 'bump' or glans attaches to a shaft about two to four centimetres long. Attached to the shaft are two clitoral 'legs' about nine to 11 centimetres long, running back into the body in a wishbone shape. Two clitoral bulbs of erectile tissue extend down to the area outside the vagina.

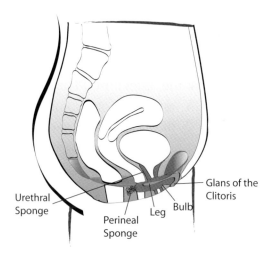

Fig. 18 - The Internal Parts of the Clitoris

Dr Helen O'Connell describes how the upper 'urethra and vagina are intimately related structures forming a tissue cluster that appears to be the locus of female sexual function and orgasm.' Women have an extensive internal sexual anatomy which is prone to damage during surgery.

During sexual arousal, the bulbs, legs, shaft and glans of the clitoris fill with blood and become firm. The PF muscles surround the legs and bulbs of the clitoris, and contract to produce the sensations of orgasm, while directing blood flow to and from the clitoris.

During orgasm, contractions start in the smooth muscles of the fallopian tubes, uterus and glands surrounding the urethra, followed by contractions of voluntary muscles located in the pelvic floor, perineum and anal sphincter. The pubococcygeus muscle contracts during orgasm, forcing blood out of erectile tissues to help create the intense sensations of orgasm.

Strong PF muscles are more responsive to arousal and contract to give the powerful sensations accompanying orgasm.

Researchers looked at the effect of PF strength exercises on sexual function in a group of women with urinary incontinence. Women in the study experiencing vaginal pain showed a marked improvement with less pain or complete relief from pain. Those with low sexual desire or difficulty achieving orgasm reported improvement in their sexual function. Women's health physiotherapists are now an integral part of treating sexual disorders in women.

Sexual arousal disorders are common when the PF muscles are over-active (too tight), with a decreased blood supply to the muscles. When intercourse is too painful to tolerate due to muscle spasms, the experience becomes distressing and impacts on the relationship. Seek assessment and early treatment to establish the cause of the pain and commence suitable treatment. To learn more: www.pelvicpain.org or www.vaginismus-awareness-network.org

Pelvic Surgery and Return to Activity

While some women report improved health and normal sexual

function after pelvic surgery, others experience an adverse effect on their sexuality.

The explanation of risks and benefits of any planned pelvic surgery should include accurate information on sexual dysfunction (decreased desire, orgasm, vaginal lubrication and pain), and be routinely discussed when surgeons gain informed consent for gynaecological surgery. With the increasing use of tape and mesh for reconstructive pelvic surgery, surgeons are reporting side effects including tape erosion and exposed mesh in the vagina. After hysterectomy, disruption of nerve supply can lead to reduced vaginal lubrication and loss of sensation with orgasm. Bladder function can be affected along with defecation problems.

Improving PF muscle control prior to surgery may help address the high rate of follow-up surgery after prolapse repair. Learning the correct PF muscle action with improved control, strength and endurance adds support for the repair post-operatively. As PF exercises are more difficult when significant prolapse is present, inserting a pessary pre-surgery to support the organs while practicing strength exercises may be more effective.

When the pelvic floor descends with coughing and activity instead of lifting, this same pattern is likely to persist post-operatively, as surgical repair does not retrain the muscles. Ongoing internal downward pressure on the surgical repair will contribute to surgical failure.

Just as urodynamic studies are commonplace prior to pelvic surgery, the same priority should be placed on identifying women who bear down or have no active lift of their pelvic floor. Retraining pelvic floor strength and abdominal muscle coordination pre-operatively is part of gaining a positive surgical result.

> *To gain full benefit from repair surgery or hysterectomy, learn and follow the guidelines for safely returning to activity after surgery.*

Before surgery, women and their partners benefit from information and written instructions about rest, bowel emptying, PF exercises, suitable activity, lifting, housework, returning to sexual activity, work and sport. Planning to have home help during the recovery time allows for uninterrupted healing after surgery.

Post-operatively, collagen strengthens the surgical site and by 60 days following surgery, the wound should achieve around 80 percent of its normal strength. The remaining 20 percent may take six months to two years to fully strengthen the surgical site.

Returning to normal activity and/or lifting more than 2-3 kilograms within six weeks of surgery, risks damage and breakdown of the surgical repair. A slow, gradual, pain free return to normal duties and sport ensures optimal healing after surgery.

Smoking slows healing post-operatively, as nicotine inhibits the formation of new blood vessels vital for healing and repair processes.

Post-operative pelvic pain and sexual dysfunction treatments include:

- soft tissue mobilisation including myofascial releases and muscle energy techniques
- postural control, breathing and relaxation techniques
- biofeedback, dilators and muscle stretches
- stabilising and strengthening exercises
- ultrasound and massage for pelvic muscle spasms

Return to Activity Guidelines

Rest

- Rest regularly during the first few weeks. Include relaxation techniques, meditation and listening to favourite music.
- Sit for short periods (20 to 30 minutes) in a straight-backed chair with lower back support. Reduce lower back strain by limiting upright sitting in bed.
- Practice postural correction by growing tall when sitting and adopting this position when sitting, standing and walking. Maintain the small inwards curve in your lower back.

Housework

- For six weeks, avoid heavier tasks such as vacuuming, grocery shopping, cleaning baths and lifting heavy washing.
- Spend 10 to 15 minutes on light duties and sit to complete tasks. Avoid a working position where your lower back is slumped.
- For six weeks, restrict gardening to picking flowers and watering with a hose.

Protecting the Sutures

- Wash the abdominal scar with a hand held shower hose and avoid using soap.
- Apply hand pressure over the scar when sneezing or coughing and lift your pelvic floor prior to the action.
- Avoid straining the surgical repair when emptying the bowel. Hold a pad firmly up over the front of the pelvic floor when the bowel opens. Take extra fibre or stool softeners, as pain medication commonly causes constipation.
- Wear a support garment.
- Avoid driving for six weeks to prevent rupture of stitches with sudden braking.
- Continue wearing compression stockings for six weeks post surgery to prevent deep vein thrombosis.
- Check with your surgeon for the 'all clear' before commencing massage around the scar with vitamin E or almond oil.

Lifting Guidelines

- Lift only two to three kilos during the first six weeks. Gradually increase activity, and stop if you feel internal strain or discomfort.
- Light duties on return to work for up to 12 weeks.
- Vary working positions between sitting and standing, always with a tall posture.
- Bend your knees and hips and keep the lower back flat instead of bending over at the waist to lift.
- Lift the pelvic floor before lifting any weight.

Exercise

- Start gentle pelvic floor exercises when the catheter and sutures are removed.
- Continue deep breathing exercises for several weeks.
- Start easy walking on level ground. By six weeks, aim to walk briskly up to four or five times per week for 30 to 40 minutes.
- Check with your surgeon for the go-ahead to start low impact exercise eg: swimming or very gentle exercise classes after eight to ten weeks. Avoid over-challenging or strenuous exercise for 6 months post surgery.
- Be cautious returning to high impact activities such as running or tennis, which should be avoided for at least 4 to 6 months.

Hygiene

- Report increased scar redness, pain, swelling, odour or oozing.
- Avoid using tampons until your surgeon gives the 'all clear'.
- Consult your doctor if fever, chills, frequency or burning occur when urinating. A mid-stream urine test will indicate the presence of infection.
- Visit a physiotherapist if you experience bowel or bladder problems, pelvic floor weakness or a sensation of heaviness.

Sexual Activity

- Check with the surgeon when it is safe to resume intercourse.

- Initally do your own vaginal wall palpation by sweeping your fingers around 360 degrees internally to check for any painful or tight areas.
- If pain is present with intercourse, see your doctor or physiotherapist.

Pain and the Pelvic Floor

Pain in the pelvis or pelvic floor is related to:

- Scar tissue from episiotomies, repair of perineal tears and adhesions after caesarean or pelvic surgery.
- Coccyx damage during birth or through falling onto the buttocks.
- Pudendal nerve damage or entrapment.
- Pelvic organ prolapse.
- Tight PF muscles with trigger points.
- Urethral diverticulum and recto-anal syndromes.
- Interstitial cystitis (inflammation of the bladder lining).
- Endometriosis which is associated with painful periods and pain during intercourse.
- A termination, pelvic cysts or chronic pelvic pain syndromes.
- Vulval pain syndrome.

Vulval pain syndrome describes various conditions causing persistant or localised pain where symptoms cause sexual dysfunction, physical and psychological distress.

Burning, throbbing or stinging sensations are felt in the vulva, along with pain and discomfort in the urethra or rectum. Vulval discomfort and pain is present with activity and in any position, limiting exercise or intercourse.

Causes of vulval pain syndrome include pelvic or vulvovaginal surgery, childbirth, injury to hips or back (eg: a herniated disc), a fall onto the buttocks, back surgery and spinal stenosis (narrowing of the canal around the spinal cord). Researchers in Boston found women who experienced pain when first using tampons were seven to eight times more likely to have vulval pain later in life. Continuing to have intercourse without arousal and in the presence of pain aggravates the condition.

Intense vulval burning can be due to trauma or entrapment of the nerves supplying the pelvic floor. Treatment includes referral to an urologist, a dermatologist (for associated skin infections) and a physiotherapist for treatment of the spine and pelvic floor.

Muscle spasms and trigger points develop in the pelvic floor and pelvic muscles when a woman walks around with continuous PF muscle tension due to pain, burning or urine loss. Overloading or excessively working a muscle causes hyperirritable trigger points generating intense local and/or referred pain to adjacent or remote body areas.

Pelvic floor physiotherapy focuses on teaching clients self treatment skills for muscle relaxation, breathing exercises, muscle stretches, soft tissue releases and suitable pelvic floor and abdominal exercises. Fibromyalgia and irritable bowel syndrome are associated chronic pain syndromes contributing to the ongoing pain and stress of vulval pain syndrome.

To learn more about vulval pain syndrome: www.nva.org or www.vulvalpainsociety.org

Taking
Action

7

Taking Action

Filling out your Personal Action Plan is the first step to success. The following pages have space to write your goals, strategies and possible barriers to success. Complete these using achievable steps to progress toward your long-term goals. Reading this book is a great start, and I encourage you to act on the information and include changes into your daily life.

Begin by -

- Completing the 'Pelvic Floor Assessment Chart' (page 148).
- Completing the 48 hour Bladder Chart (page 149) to gain an overview of how frequently you pass urine and the amount voided.
- Completing The 7-Day Bowel Chart (page 150) gives an overview of your bowel frequency, control and stool consistency.
- Discuss the results from the three charts with your doctor or womens health physiotherapist.
- Complete your Personal Action Plan, starting on page 151 to record your pelvic floor goals, the habits you wish to change and the new habits to adopt.
- Read this action plan regularly to ensure you stay on course.

Pelvic Floor Assessment Chart

Complete the following responses and take the completed chart to your doctor if 'yes' answers are recorded.

Bladder	No	Yes
Do you lose urine with sneezing or exercising?		
Does urgency cause frequent voiding?		
Do you lose urine due to sudden urgency?		
Do you empty more than 6 times daily?		
At night, do you get up more than once to empty?		
Do you lose urine at night in bed?		
Have you stopped exercising due to urine loss?		
Is urine loss affecting your quality of life?		
Bowel		
Does your bowel empty more than 3 times per day?		
Does your bowel empty less than twice per week?		
Do you have difficulty controlling wind?		
Do you occasionally lose bowel matter?		
Do you strain to empty your bowel?		
Do you have haemorrhoids or anal fissures?		
Is it difficult to fully empty your bowel?		
Intimacy		
Do you have pain with intercourse?		
Has vaginal sensation with intercourse altered?		
Is your orgasm less intense?		
Prolapse		
Does your pelvic floor feel 'heavier' at end of day?		
Do you have a bulge at your vaginal entrance?		
Do you experience abdominal or back pain?		
Count the total 'Yes' answers:		

Hold it Sister 48 Hour Bladder Chart

Date	Time	Vol (ml)	Pad Status	Pad Change	Fluid Intake
12 Sep	6.05am	550	N/A	N/A	300ml water
	9.45am	240	Damp	YES	250ml coffee
Total Output			**Total Intake**		

Pad Status: dry/damp/wet/soaked
Pad Change: Did you change pad? Yes or No (N/A if not using pads)
Fluid Intake – list all consumed

Hold It Sister 7 Day Bowel Chart

Date	Time	Urgency	Loss type	Strain to open	Pain	Blood	Consistency & shape
4 Jun	2pm	No	W	Yes	rectum	Yes	Hard, lumpy
7 Jun	8am	Yes	L	No	No	No	Loose, pebbles

Urgency   Feeling of marked urgency? Yes / No
Loss   Involuntary loss of **S**olid, **L**iquid, **M**ucous or **W**ind – or None
Strain   Difficulty emptying / manual assistance – Yes / No

Pain   Yes / No – if yes, note location
Bleeding   Yes / No
Consistency eg: hard/loose/watery
Shape   eg: sausage/pebbles/lumpy

Personal Action Plan

My Pelvic Floor Goals

(Examples: To exercise without leaking, control my urgent bladder, sit and stand tall.)

_____

_____

_____

_____

_____

_____

_____

_____

_____

_____

_____

_____

_____

_____

_____

_____

Damaging Pelvic Floor Habits To Change

(Examples: Stop slumping when I sit, retrain my upper chest breathing pattern, add more fibre, use new toilet position to avoid straining, or relax tight waist muscles.)

_____

_____

_____

_____

_____

_____

_____

_____

_____

_____

_____

_____

_____

_____

_____

My New Pelvic Floor Habits

(Examples: I will eat five serves of vegetables and two serves of fruit daily to soften my poo, I will learn PF exercises and make them a part of my daily routine.)

_____

_____

_____

_____

_____

_____

_____

_____

_____

_____

_____

_____

_____

_____

_____

_____

Resources

Physiotherapists & Continence Organisations Call the
Physiotherapy Association in your state or province.

- Ask your local physiotherapist, doctor, community health nurse, gynaecologist or pharmacist for the name of a local women's health physiotherapist.

- Call the Continence Foundation for the contact details of a women's health physiotherapist in your area.

Physiotherapy Associations

Australian Physiotherapy Association
www.physiotherapy.asn.au   Tel: 03 90920888

New Zealand Physiotherapy Association
www.physiotherapy.org.nz   Tel: 64 4801 6500

Singapore Physiotherapy Association
www.physiotherapy.org.sg

U.K. Physiotherapy Association
www.csp.org.uk   Tel: 020 7306 6666

U.S.A. Physical Therapy Association
www.apta.org   Tel: 8009992782

Canadian Physiotherapy Association
www.thesehands.ca   Tel: 1 800 387 8679

Irish Society of Chartered Physiotherapists
www.iscp.ie   Tel: +35 314022148

Netherlands Physiotherapy Association
www.fysionet.nl   Tel: +0 3346 72 900

Continence Organisations

Australian Continence Foundation
www.continence.org.au   Tel: 1800 33 00 66

N.Z. Continence Association
www.continence.org.nz   Tel: 0800 650 659

Singapore Continence Association
www.sfcs.org.sg   Tel: +65 6787 0337

U.K. Bladder & Bowel Foundation
www.bladderandbowelfoundation.org   Tel: 0845 345 0165

U.S.A. Continence Association
www.nafc.org   Tel: 1 800 252 3337

Canadian Continence Association
www.continence-fdn.ca   Tel: 705 750-4600

Irish Continence Society
www.continence.ie

World Federation of Incontinence Patients.
www.wfip.org

Worldwide Continence Organization
www.continenceworldwide.org

References

Section 1 The Pelvic Floor

Elneil S. 2007 Vesico-Vaginal & Recto-Vaginal fistula in the developing world. ICS News, Issue 5 January 2007, International Continence Society.

Hagen et al. 2004. Conservative management of pelvic organ prolapse in women. The Cochrane Database of Systematic Reviews, http://www.cochrane.org/reviews/en/ab003882.html.

Bai SW, Jeon MJ, Kim JY, Chung KA, Kim SK, and Park KH. 2002. Relationship between stress urinary incontinence and pelvic organ prolapse. Int Urogyn J.13(4):256-260.

De Lancey J. 2005. The hidden epidemic of pelvic floor dysfunction. J.American Journal of Ob. & Gyn. 192(5),1488-1495.

Meyer S., Hohlfeld P., et al. 2001. Birth trauma: short and long term effects of forceps delivery compared with spontaneous delivery on various pelvic floor parameters. BJOG 107(11): 1360-1370.

Burgio KL, Brubaker L, Richter H et al. 2010 Patient satisfaction with stress incontinence surgery. J Neurourol Urodyn 29(8):1403-09

Hodges PW 2006. Low back pain and the pelvic floor. In: The Pelvic Floor, Carriere B. & Markel-Zeldt C (Eds), Thieme, Stuttgart.

Kiff ES, Barnes PR, Swash M. 1984. Evidence of pudendal neuropathy in patients with perineal descent and chronic straining at stool. Gut 25:1279-1282.

Subak, LL. 2009 Weight loss to treat urinary incontinence in overweight and obese women. NEJM 360(5):481-490

Hunskaar S. 2008. A systematic review of overweight and obesity as risk factors and targets for clinical intervention for urinary incontinence in women. J Neurourol Urodyn 27(8):749-757

Maserejian NN, Giovannucci EL, McVary KT, McGrother C & McKinlay JB. 2010. Dietary macronutrient and energy intake and urinary incontinence in women. Am J Epidemiol. 171(10):1116-1125

Subak LL, Johnson C, Johnson C, Whitcomb E, Boban D, Saxton J. and Brown JS, 2002. Does weight loss improve incontinence in moderately obese women? Inter Urogyn J.(2002) 13(1):40-43

Norton P, Baker J, Sharp H, Warenski J. 1995. Genitourinary prolapse and joint hypermobility in women. Obstet Gynecol. 85(2):225-8

Bo K, Fleten C, Nystad W. 2009. Effect of antenatal pelvic floor muscle training on labor and birth. Obstet Gynecol. 113(6):1279-84

Hoff Braekken I, Majida M, Engh M, Bo K. 2011. Morphological changes after pelvic floor muscle training measured by 3D ultrasonography: a randomised controlled trial. Obstet Gynecol

Section 2 Pelvic Floor Habits

Markwell S. 1998. Functional disorders of the anorectum and pain syndromes. In: Women's Health: A textbook for physiotherapists, Sapsford R. Bullock-Saxton J. and Markwell S. (Eds) WB Saunders Co. London p.357

Jorgsen S, Hein HO and Gyntelberg F. 1994. Heavy lifting at work and risk of genital prolapse and herniated lumbar disc in assistant nurses. Occup Med 44:47-49.

Woodman PJ, Swift SE, O'Boyle AL, Valley MT, Bland DR, Kahn MA and Schaffer JI. 2006. Prevalence of severe pelvic organ prolapse in relation to job description and socioeconomic status: a multicentre cross-sectional study. Int Urogyn J. 17(4):340-345

Smith, MD, Coppieters MW, et al. 2007. Postural response of the pelvic floor and abdominal muscles in women with and without incontinence. Neuro Urodyn 26(3): 377-385.

Section 3 Training the Pelvic Floor

Hodges PW 2006. Low back pain and the pelvic floor. In: The Pelvic Floor, Carriere B. & Markel-Zeldt C (Eds), Thieme, Stuttgart.

Kegel AH, 1948. The non surgical treatment of genital relaxation, West, Med & Surg. 31:213-216.

Section 4 Activity and the Pelvic Floor

Nygaard IE, Thompson FL, Svengalis SL and Albright JP. 1994. Urinary incontinence in elite nulliparous athletes. Obstet Gynecol 84:183-187).

Thyssen HH, Clevin L, Olesen S, Lose G. 2002. Urinary incontinence in elite female athletes and dancers. Int Urogyn J. 13(1):15-17

Bo K. Borgen JS. 2001. Prevalence of stress and urge urinary incontinence in elite athletes and controls. Med Sci Sports Ex. 33(11):1797-1802.

Eliasson K, Larsson T, Mattsson E. 2002. Prevalence of stress incontinence in nulliparous elite trampolinists. Scand J of Med & Sci in Sports 12(2):106-110.

Eliasson K, Edner A, Mattsson E. 2008. Urinary incontinence in very young and mostly nulliparous women with a history of organised high-impact trampoline training: occurrence and risk factors. Int Urogyn J 19(5):687-696.

Salvesen K, Mørkved S. Randomised controlled trial of pelvic floor muscle training during pregnancy. BMJ. 2004 August 14; 329(7462): 378–380.

Boissonnault J, Blaschak M. Incidence of diastasis recti abdominis during the childbearing year. Physical Therapy 1988;68:1082-1086

Spitznagel T, Leong F, Van Dillen L. Prevelance of diastasis recti Abdominis in a urogynaelogical population. Int Urogyn J. 2007Vol 18(3):321-328

Dudding TC, Vaizey CJ, Kamm MA. Obstetric anal sphincter injury: incidence, risk factors, and management. Ann Surg. 2008 Feb;247(2):224-37.

Matzel K, Manuel Besendörfer M, Kuschel S. The Anal Sphincter. Pelvic floor education .2008, Part V, 289-292, DOI: 10.1007/978-1-84628-505-9_36

Altomare DF, Ratto C, Ganio E, Lolli P, Masin A, Villani RD. Long-term outcome of sacral nerve stimulation for fecal incontinence. Dis Colon Rectum. 2009;52(1):11-7.

Section 5 Pregnancy, Birth and Postpartum

Beckmann, M, Garrett A. 2006. Antenatal perineal massage for reducing perineal trauma. Cochrane Database Syst Rev. Jan 25(1):CD005123.

Fynes M. 2003. Effect of pregnancy and delivery on post vaginal compartment. Proceedings, Int Continence Society 33rd Annual Meeting Florence.

De Tayrac R, Panel L, Masson G. and Mares P. 2006. Episiotomy and prevention of perineal and pelvic floor injuries. J Gyn Obst Biol Reprod (Paris) 2006 Feb;35(1 Suppl):1S24-1S31).

Signorello LB, Harlow BL, Chekos, AK and Repke JT. 2001. Postpartum sexual functioning and its relationship to perineal trauma: a retrospective cohort study of primiparous women. Am J Obstet Gynecol.184(5):881-8.

Dietz HP, Hyland G and Hay-Smith J. 2006. The assessment of levator trauma: A comparison between palpation and 4D pelvic floor ultrasound Neurourol Urodyn 25(5):424-427.

Jack GS, Kikolova G, Vilain E, Raz S, Rodriguez L. 2006. Familial transmission of genitovaginal prolapse. .Int Urogyn J. 17(5):498-501.

Sakala C. 2006. Comparing harms of vaginal and Caesarian birth: Maternity Centre Association's Systematic Review and Education and Quality Improvement Campaign. Childbirth Connection http://www.childbirthconnection.org/article.asp?ck=10271&ClickedLink=200&area=2.

Serati M, Salvatore S, Uccella S, Nappi R, Bolis P. 2009. Female urinary incontinence during intercourse: a review on an understudied problem for women's sexuality. J Sex Med. Jan;6(1):40-48

Sneddon A, Ellwood D. 2004. Post Partum Care. Australian Doctor, April 30, 2004: p40.

Wesnes SL, Huskaar S, Bo K, Rortveit G. 2010. Urinary incontinence and weight change during pregnancy and postpartum: a cohort study. Am J Epidemiol. 172(9):1034-44

Bo K. 2009. Does pelvic floor muscle training prevent and treat urinary and fecal incontinence in pregnancy? Nat Clin Pract Urol 6(3):122-123

Hay-Smith J, Morkved S, Fairbrother K, Hergison G. 2009. Pelvic floor muscle training for prevention and treatment of urinary and faecal incontinence in ante natal and post natal women. Evid Based Med. 14(2):53

Morkved S, Bo K, Schei B, Salvesen KA. 2003 Pelvic floor muscle training during pregnancy to prevent urinary incontinence: a single blind randomized controlled tiral. O&G 101:131-319

Boissonnault J, Blaschak M. Incidence of diastasis recti abdominis during the childbearing year. Physical Therapy 1988;68:1082-1086

Spitznagel T, Leong F, Van Dillen L. Prevelance of diastasis recti Abdominis in a urogynaelogical population. Int Urogyn J. 2007Vol 18(3):321-328

Viktrup L, Rortveit G, Lose G. Risk of stress urinary incontinence 12 years after the first pregnancy and delivery. O&G 2006;108(2):248-254.

Section 6 Menopause and the Pelvic Floor

Smith DB, A continence care approach for long term care facilities. Geriatric Nursing. Vol 19, Issue 2.81-86

Jackson SL, Boyko EJ. And Fihn SD. 2005. Urinary incontinence and diabetes in postmenopausal women. Diab. Care 28(7):17301738.

Smith DB. 2006. Urinary incontinence and diabetes: a review. J.Wound Ostomy & Cont. Nurs. 33(6):619-23.

Knowler WC, Barrett-Connor E, Fowler SE, Hamman RF, Lachin JM, Walker EA and Nathan DM. 2002. Reduction in the incidence of type-2 diabetes with lifestyle intervention or Metformin. New Eng. J.Med. 346(6):393-403.

Haylen B.T. 2006. The retroverted prolapse: ignored to date but core to prolapse. Inter Urogyn J. 17(6):555-558.

How common is pelvic organ prolapse(and is this a normal finding)? Medscape Ob/Gyn&Womens Health Report from 24th annual meeting of AUGS http://www.medscape.com/viewarticle/461719_7.

Fernando RJ. Thakar R. Sultan AH. 2006. Are vaginal pessaries as effective as surgery in symptomatic pelvic organ prolapse? 31st Annual Int Urogyn. Assoc. Meeting, Athens, Greece, 6-9 Sept 2006.

Avorn J, Monane M, Gurwitz JH, Glynn RJ, Choodnovskiy I, Lipsitz LA.et al.1994. Reduction of bacteriuria and pyuria after ingestion of cranberry juice. JAMA, 271(10);751-754.

Stanford EJ and McMurphy C. 2006. There is a low incidence of bladder bacteriuria in painful bladder syndrome/interstitial cystitis patients followed longitudinally. Int Urogyn J. 17(Sup 2):S85.

Koch PB, Mansfield PK, Thurau D, Carey M. 2005. Feeling Frumpy: the relationships between body image and sexual response changes in midlife women. J of Sex Res. 42(3):215-223.

Northrup C. 2003. The Wisdom of Menopause. Bantam, New York.

Hunskaar S 2006. State-of-the-art address. Proceedings of I.C.S. 36th Annual Meeting. Christchurch.

Northrup C. 2008. The Secret Pleasures of Menopause. Hay House, New York.

Rogers R. Report from the 24th annual meeting of AUGS. Med Gen Med e-Journal, http://www.medscape.com/viewarticle/461719_6.

Trimbos JB, Maas CP, Deruiter MC, Peters AAW, Kenter GG. 2001. A nerve-sparing radical hysterectomy: Guidelines and feasibility in western patients. Int J Gynecol Cancer 11(3):180-186.

Roovers JPWR, Raart CH van der. 2006. Damage to vaginal innervation is more extensive during vaginal prolapse surgery than during abdominal prolapse surgery. Int Urogyn J. 17(Sup 2):S74.

Maxwell D. 2004. Surgical Techniques in Obstetrics and Gynaecology. Churchill Livingstone, New York.

Harlow B. and Gunther-Stewart E. 2003. A population-based assessment of chronic unexplained vulvar pain: have we underestimated the prevalence of vulvodynia? JAMWA. 58(2):82-88.

Travell J. & Simons D. 1983. Myofascial pain and Dysfunction: The trigger point manual. Williams &Wilkins, Baltimore MD

Wise D., Anderson, R. 2008. A Headache In The Pelvis: a new understanding and treatment for chronic pelvic pain syndromes. 5th Ed. National Centre for Pelvic Pain Research, Occidental, California,

Gittes R., Nakamura, M. 1996. Female Urethral Syndrome - a female prostatitis? West J Med 164:435-438

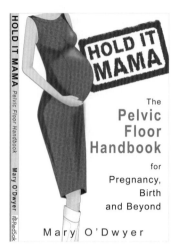

Mary O'Dwyer's new book Hold It Mama is an indispensible guide to the pelvic floor, pelvis and abdomen during pregnancy, birth and postpartum.

This long awaited book guides readers on preventing and healing specific problems before, during and following birth. It is filled with expert advice and exercises to recover dynamic stability after vaginal and caesarean births.

Like many pregnancies, this remarkable book is well overdue!

Available from August 2011 at all leading Australian bookstores and soon after in the UK. Order online at www.holditsister.com or www.incostress.com (UK only).

To receive Mary's monthly newsletter, register email at www.holditsister.com

To enquire about Mary's workshops or book her as a speaker, contact admin@redsok.com

Hold it Sister